Accident and Emergency

Jane Barrett
SRN, RN(USA), RCNT, DipN, RNT
Tutor, School of Nursing
Selly Oak Hospital
Birmingham

Blackwell Scientific Publications
Oxford London Edinburgh
Boston Melbourne

© 1983 by
Blackwell Scientific Publications
Editorial offices:
Osney Mead, Oxford OX2 0EL
8 John Street, London WC1N 2ES
9 Forrest Road, Edinburgh EH1 2QH
52 Beacon Street, Boston,
　Massachusetts 02108 USA
99 Barry Street, Carlton, Victoria
　3053 Australia

All rights reserved. No part of this
publication may be reproduced,
stored in a retrieval system, or
transmitted, in any form or by any
means, electronic, mechanical,
photocopying, recording or
otherwise without the prior
permission of the copyright owner

First published 1983

Set by Burns & Smith, Derby

Printed and bound by
Billing and Sons Ltd, Worcester

Distributors

USA
　Blackwell Mosby Book Distributors
　11830 Westline Industrial Drive
　St Louis. Missouri 63141

Canada
　Blackwell Mosby Book Distributors
　120 Melford Drive, Scarborough
　Ontario M1B 2X4

Australia
　Blackwell Scientific Book Distributors
　214 Berkeley Street, Carlton
　Victoria 3053

British Library
Cataloguing in Publication Data

Barrett, Jane
　Accident and emergency nursing.
　1. Emergency nursing
　I. Title
　610.73'61　　　RT120.E4

ISBN 0-632-00958-6.

Contents

Foreword, vii

Preface, viii

Acknowledgements, x

1 The Accident and Emergency Department, 1
2 Reception and Assessment of the Patient, 20
3 Emergency Assessment and Management, 38
4 Minor Injuries, 61
5 Cardiac Emergencies, 106
6 Acute Respiratory Conditions, 131
7 Disturbances in Skin Function and Body Surface Trauma, 142
8 The Unconscious Patient, 155
9 Bone and Soft Tissue Trauma and Plastering, 195
10 Surgical and Gynaecological Emergencies, 261
11 Violence and Major Disasters, 275

Bibliography, 285

Index, 286

Foreword

The accident and emergency department is, in effect, the 'front door' of any hospital but so often the Cinderella in many ways. Its equipment is frequently obsolete or obsolescent, overworked and badly handled. Because of increasing demand, extensions and improvisations have not enhanced the facilities. Room is at a premium; patients appear in an unending flow with the whole gamut of trivia and human tragedy. Despite all this, "casualty departments" often handle more patients than the average "outpatients' department" in the parent hospital. Frequently overworked, these units manage cheerfully to give satisfaction to patient and staff alike.

Because of her knowledge gained in such busy departments, Miss Barrett has produced an invaluable reference manual for nurses coming into the department for the first time and for other workers who need a refresher in their techniques. The nurse, whose previous training has been in the relative calm of the school or ward, is often overwhelmed by this first experience of primary care. It is the nurse who has the first contact with the patient, anxious or frightened, with relatives unable to think or act rationally because of fear. This manual will give the nurses a reference book answering most of the problems likely to be faced in the average accident and emergency department, thus helping them to overcome feelings of inadequacy.

Miss Barrett emphasizes throughout the whole aspect of relationship with patient and relatives associated with the highest technical training and the importance of continuous communication. Just as someone is welcomed with attentive politeness at the front door of a home, so should the nurse deal with the worried person in the accident and emergency department.

The nurses have a very privileged position since they are much closer to the patients than anyone else. They do 'things' for the patient and the physical contact is most important.

T.W.B.Cull
MB, ChB, MRCS, LRCP

Formerly Clinical Tutor
Accident and Emergency Department
Selly Oak Hospital

Preface

The need for this book was indicated by the popularity of a small booklet about bandaging which was designed for the use of nurses and nurse learners working in the accident and emergency departments.

Interest was particularly shown in the clarity of the booklet's illustrations as well as in its emphasis upon explanations which have helped nurses both to apply bandages appropriately and to instruct patients to take over management of their own dressings. For this reason, the present book incorporates the booklet and deals with many of the tasks in a similar way which may confront nurses and nurse learners on their initiation into the work of an accident and emergency department. Although this book's main concern is to describe nursing procedures and care, related aspects of anatomy and physiology are included, which I feel will make this book useful to the nurse training for State enrollment, State registration and especially the nurses on the Joint Board Courses, Nos. 210 and 198 involved with accident and emergency work. I also feel this will be a useful book for ambulance personnel on the A.E.M.T. course, as their training includes anatomy and physiology related to disease and injuries and the initial care of a patient on entering the hospital. One of the problems in departments is the variety of experience and approaches to nursing treatment: it is hoped that nurse learners and the nursing staff will make use of this book as a basis for teaching and learning.

Many nurses are apprehensive about working in the accident and emergency department. I would hope this book will allay some of the fears, expecially the fear of the unknown, by providing basic knowledge for the nurse. For this reason, when possible, I would suggest that the nurse reads various sections before commencement of work within the department. These sections are:

The role of the nurse
Reception of the patient
Assessment of the patient
General treatment of the patient
Care of minor injuries

The remaining sections of the book deal with more specific problems which will be invariably encountered, e.g. the patient with an acute heart condition or the unconscious patient, etc. It is hoped that those reading these sections will gain a deeper understanding of the patient's condition and treatment; it is also hoped that alongside this deeper understanding will grow a sense of the excitement and satisfaction to be gained from being able to take action when and how it is demanded.

I have specifically written this book with the nurse in mind that is why in some sections the emphasis is on the nurse's responsibilities. The section on the recording of an electrocardiogram is an example. This is not a nursing responsibility, as yet, the nurse may assist the doctor or even at times take a recording for the doctor. It is, however, the doctor's responsibility to interpret the reading and prescribe the treatment. I explain how the abnormalities recorded on an electrocardiogram are also demonstrated in blood pressure and pulse observations which are the nurse's responsibility. To enable the doctor to record an electrocardiogram the nurse may connect the electrodes to the patient, as shown in the book. Another procedure, intubation, (the passing of an endotrachial tube) again is not a nurse's responsibility, but the nurse must assist the anaesthetist.

Obstetric patients come to the Accident and Emergency department often with a complication of their pregnancy in which case they require the care of trained personnel. In this section my emphasis is on summoning the appropriate help immediately and then preparing equipment that might be needed.

This book has also been written with consideration to some aspects of training the nurse will have already received and with the variety of hospital procedures in mind. I do not feel it is necessary to give the cardiac arrest procedure in detail, instead I have discussed the principles of the procedure and emphasized that you must know your own hospital procedure. Again hospital procedures can vary, e.g. care of the patient's property, or in the event of a major disaster. That is why this book is intended as a guide to the nurse — the how and the why — of accident and emergency care.

Jane Barrett   Birmingham 1983

Acknowledgements

I would like to acknowledge the help of many people concerned with the production of this book. Special thanks to Smith and Nephew for letting me incorporate the material from their original booklet on pages 241-60. The initial booklet was produced with assistance from Sister J. Little and Sister Finnegan with diagrams compiled by Mr M. Taylor. I would like to thank Mr J.J. Wood DNE for his suggestion to send the booklet for publication which started this book.

My thanks go to my colleagues Mrs C. Cason, Mrs M. Ridley and Mrs R. Natrajan for their helpful guidance and correction. Also thanks to Dr Cull and to Dr J.A. Finnegan MB, ChB, MRCP for his assistance with neurological facts. My especial thanks go to Mrs N.P. Barrett for coping with the typing of the manuscript and to Mr I. Barrett for his excellent work in completing the diagrams for this book.

Continued thanks go to Miss P. Holbrook of Blackwell Scientific Publications firstly for her faith in the fact that the book could be completed and secondly for her guidance throughout, and to Miss G. Campbell for her editorial work and the production department for the work from manuscript to bound book.

1
The Accident and Emergency Department

The accident and emergency department is the entrance to the hospital for all medical and surgical emergencies, varying from major to minor conditions. It is the entrance through which many patients come unexpectedly and sometimes unwillingly.

FUNCTION

Basically, the function of the department is to provide a high standard of care for all patients following an accident or emergency situation. As the conditions vary so widely, accident and emergency nursing is an interesting and stimulating challenge.

As the work of the department is so broad it demands staff with a diversity of skills working closely together. Working within, or available to, the department will be doctors from the different specialities, nursing staff both trained and in training, auxiliary staff, social workers and porters. The nurse in an accident and emergency department needs, therefore, to communicate with many people. However, the work of the nurse is mainly to anticipate and to meet the needs of:
    The patient
    The doctor
    The relative

The needs of the patient which the nurses and doctors aim to meet are those which are compatible with life and health. No two patients have the same needs which means that the medical and nursing staff learn to adapt their care to the requirements of each individual patient covering all physical and psychological aspects.

ATTENDANCE

The types of patient who attend an accident and emergency department can be divided into two groups. They are those who:
    Bring themselves or are brought by a relative or friend to the hospital.
    Come by ambulance to the hospital, i.e., emergency or '999' patients.

Reason

The reason why patients attend the hospital may be due to:
    An accident
    A medical or surgical emergency
    A referral to the hospital by their general practitioner.
Other factors which influence the decision as to which hospital patients attend:
    It is the local hospital.
    They have been patients in this hospital before.

Possible Outcome

The possible outcome of attending an accident and emergency department may mean that the patient is:
Treated in the department and discharged home with a follow-up appointment with the general practitioner or district nurse.
Treated in the department and then referred to other medical services for a follow-up visit, e.g., from a health visitor.
Referred in the department to a specialist doctor within the hospital with the view that treatment will require admission to hospital.

THE ROLE OF THE NURSE

The role of the nurse in the accident and emergency department is to be active and alert to the needs of those within the department and ready to make full use of all skills wherever and whenever they are demanded. A nurse in the accident and emergency department has a vital and extremely varied part to play. A nurse must:

Be aware at all times of the needs of the patient.
Assess each patient first as care must be related to the patient's condition and the urgency of treatment.
Assist the doctor in examinations, investigations and treatments.
Know the location of all equipment to be able to give proper assistance.
One of the first responsibilities of a nurse coming into the department is to become familiar with the layout and with all functional aspects of the department.

Departmental Layout

Most accident and emergency departments are basically laid out in the same way. Usually there are two separate entrances; one entrance for walk-in patients and one for ambulance patients. The walk-in patients will be registered at the reception desk and stay in the waiting room until shown to a cubicle where they generally sit for treatment. The ambulance patient is taken directly into the department and transferred from the ambulance chair or stretcher to a hospital trolley in a cubicle.

Each accident and emergency department has a special area for dealing with an emergency. This may vary from a small cubicle to a room capable of containing 4 patients. The position of this area varies in each department; in some the room is next to the entrance while in others it is right inside the department. The nurse must know where the area is, be aware when a patient is in the area and must respond to assist in care.

Most departments have their own sterile areas (theatres) and these are used for an assortment of procedures. Asepsis is an essential part of the treatment for many injuries. It is important to be able to distinguish infected wounds from clean injuries, although both require aseptic conditions they will not be treated in the same area due to the possible risk of cross-infection.

Nurses need to learn the layout of their particular department on their first day and begin to locate equipment, using any free time during the day to investigate the contents of the storage cupboards. The equipment (Figure 1) which must be easily located includes:
Emergency equipment
Defibrillator

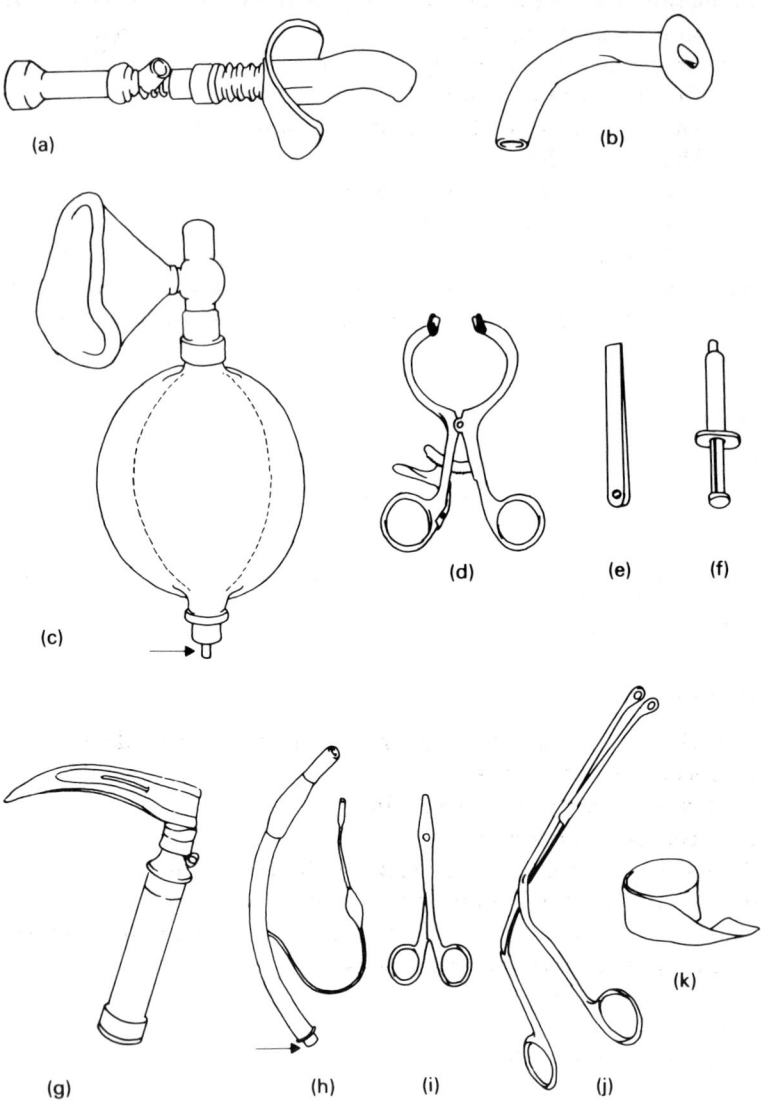

Figure 1 Emergency equipment: Brook's airway (a); Guedal airway (b); Ambu bag, with face mask (c), **Note** connection (indicated by arrow) for oxygen supply; mouth gag (d); wooden wedge (e); syringe, for injecting air into endotracheal tube (f); laryngoscope (g); endotracheal tube, of appropriate size (h), **Note** connection (indicated by arrow) for use with Ambu bag; Spencer Wells artery forceps (i); Magill forceps (j); bandage to secure endotracheal tube in place (k).

Suction apparatus and oxygen — making sure you know how
to use this equipment.
Drug cupboards including:
Control drug cupboard
Drugs used to neutralize poisons *(antidotes)*
Drugs used for:
Cardiac arrest (see Chapter 5)
Epilepsy (see Chapter 8)
Diabetes (see Chapter 8)
The patients' trolleys used in accident and emergency units differ and the nurse must be familiar with the operation of each type.

Assessment

To assess a patient's condition the nurse must be aware of the location of the appropriate equipment:
Sphygmomanometer
Stethoscope
Thermometer
Charts for recording results

Investigation

For the investigation or examination which the doctor will perform, the nurse must:
1 Prepare the patient accordingly.
2 Prepare the equipment.
3 Assist the doctor to perform the investigation.
4 Clear away the equipment after use.
The nurse must when necessary locate the equipment for the following diagnostic investigations:
The taking of blood samples
Rectal examinations
Vaginal examination
Neurological examination
Examination of urine including routine test and midstream urine.

General Responsibilities

While working in an accident and emergency department, a nurse must become proficient in procedures which may vary

The Accident and Emergency Department   5

slightly from one hospital to another. Those procedures which involve treatment of the patient are:
Care of minor injuries.
Assisting with suturing.
Preparation for a general anaesthetic.
Assisting or performing a gastric lavage.
Assisting with the erection of an intravenous infusion.
Administration of drugs including preparation and recording. Drugs given in the accident and emergency department, as all other drugs, must be recorded at the time of administration in the correct place.
Application of skin traction.
Application of a Thomas' splint.

The nurse may be required to catheterize a female patient to obtain a urine specimen and to assist the doctor if a male patient is to be catheterized. Other responsibilities of the nurse include care of:
The patient's belongings and valuables.
Relatives or friends, notifying them if necessary.
The infectious or infected patient.

The final responsibility of the nurse is to:
The discharged patient — to give instructions verbally and in writing regarding future care.
The patient who requires admission to hospital. Ensure that the ward is prepared to receive the patient and that the ward staff are given the following information:
1   The patient's name, age and diagnosis.
2   The treatment already given in the accident and emergency department.
3   The treatment which the patient is to receive in the ward.
4   Whether the next of kin has been informed.

Before leaving the department the nurse who escorts a patient to the ward must ensure that all this information accompanies the patient.

Communication

Communication is vital for nurses to be able to perform their role properly and efficiently. They will communicate with patients, ambulance personnel, doctors and the patient's relatives or friends.

Patients

Communication with patients immediately on admission and while preparing them for the doctor's examination is essential. Although patients will need to give information related to the injury or condition to the doctor, asking questions and talking to the nurse can initially:

Make patients feel that someone is interested in their condition and is taking care of them.

Allow the nurse to discover any relevant facts about the patients that should be conveyed to the doctor to assist in the diagnosis or treatment.

Patients do not always give the nurse and the doctor the same information. Another important factor in this interchange is the relief of anxiety. The nurse is often able to give explanations and reassurance to patients during this initial communication. For example, a patient may be extremely distressed by pain and may assume that this indicates some serious illness. Asking the patient to describe the pain and assuring the patient that it is to be expected under the circumstances can relieve undue anxiety. Possibly the patient who has fallen and complains of pain in the buttock may only have this pain because of a bruise, and this explanation may help the patient to relax. The bruise, however, does not rule out further injury which must, of course, be investigated. This leads to another form of concern for the patient. Some patients feel that they are in the department under false pretences, their injury or illness seems trivial to them. Each patient must be encouraged to feel that his or her case is important and worthy of investigation. 'Casual' treatment of any patient is unprofessional .

Ambulance Personnel

Ambulance personnel should communicate with a senior nurse in the department and explain the patient's present condition. It is essential to obtain an accurate report on the patient as this will indicate:

The immediacy of required treatment.
How the patient should be moved and positioned.
The surrounding circumstances of the incident.
Any relevant care or treatment required.

Doctors

Communication with doctors includes any information obtained from the patient or ambulance personnel. Further communication will occur during the treatment of the patient.

Relatives

Relatives (or the accompanying friend) must be informed of the patient's condition and also their subsequent role in the care of the patient.

Further Responsibilities

Further responsibilities involve communicating with other personnel either inside or outside the department (Figure 2). Patient information is always confidential so if anything is imparted by the nurse it must be concerned with the patient's care.

Nurse	Nurse and Doctor	Doctor
Porters	Patient	Police
Ward staff	Relative	Hospital administration
Social worker	Other nursing and	Newspaper reporters
District nurse	medical staff	

Figure 2 Lines of communication inside and outside the department showing that although nurses and doctors communicate with the same people, they also have the separate responsibility of communicating with specific people.

As the nurse is responsible for the co-ordination of care, communication with other health workers is another responsibility.

The doctor must have all information needed to refer to other doctors for second opinions, and may be involved with speaking to the police. In most departments police matters are discussed directly between the police and the patient providing the doctor thinks that the patient is in a fit condition and the patient consents.

Newspaper reporters should be referred to the hospital administrator.

General Advice

General advice for a nurse beginning work in an accident and emergency department is:
1   It will take about a week before you feel you know your way about the department.
2   There may be an initial feeling of inadequacy — this is quite common but will soon pass as you begin to have some experience and to become proficient in some care.
3   The accident and emergency department will not be as organized as a ward. The nature of its work means that no one can predict the quiet or the busy times so learn to accept this and adjust to the priorities.
4   Remember other staff will help you so ask them if you have any questions, even if it is sometimes the same question. Everything cannot be remembered at once and it is wiser to make sure.
5   The accident and emergency department provides many experiences, learn from all of them. Ask to observe procedures if staff numbers permit and participate in care when requested. Ask about any care or treatment. In some instances teaching can be carried out at the time of the incident to the benefit of both patient and nurse learner. However, if care is urgent and time does not allow for teaching, ask about factors which are not understood at a later time.

As a nurse learner be prepared to ask questions of the doctors as well; when circumstances permit, they are only too willing to teach. The important point is to take every opportunity to learn, whether as a nurse learner or as a new staff member. Remember that each patient in the accident and emergency department is unique, and you may see a particular condition or treatment only once in your nursing career.
6   As a nurse learner or new staff coming into the accident and emergency department you may be apprehensive but remember there is always qualified, competent staff on hand to help and advise. So be inquisitive, accept the challenge and enjoy working in the accident and emergency department.

Lifting and Moving

Lifting and moving the acutely ill patient incorrectly without sufficient knowledge of the injury can cause the patient further injury. Remember the words of Florence Nightingale: 'The hospital should do the patient no harm'.

Before moving any patient the nurse must first **Stop** and **Think quickly.**

Be aware of the urgency of moving the patient but find out what is wrong. Acutely ill patients are generally brought to the hospital by ambulance personnel who can give a quick brief history from which priorities can be set. Allow the ambulance personnel to lift the patient onto the hospital trolley as they are aware of the patient's injuries. Assist them when necessary. Ambulance personnel can lift the patient either manually or with the aid of poles and a stretcher canvas or a scoop stretcher.

If the patient requires resuscitation then the lifting onto a trolley should be carried out quickly and resuscitation commenced.

Before Lifting

Before lifting it is important to:
1   Stop — Think.
2   Assess the patient's injuries.
3   Decide on appropriate movement.
4   Summon enough help.
5   Ensure that the patient is placed on a suitable trolley for the injuries, e.g., hard surface for a fracture.

While Lifting

While lifting ensure that the:
1   Patient's airway is maintained (Figure 3).
2   Fractures are immmobilized. The correct care of fractures is vital and is detailed in Chapter 9.

Once the patient is lifted onto the trolley, then he or she must be put into a position suitable for the injury.

The 3 main nursing positions referred to in this book and shown in Figure 3 are:

    Recumbent — flat on the back with one or no pillows.

    Semirecumbent — on back but propped up with several pillows.

    Semiprone — on one side.

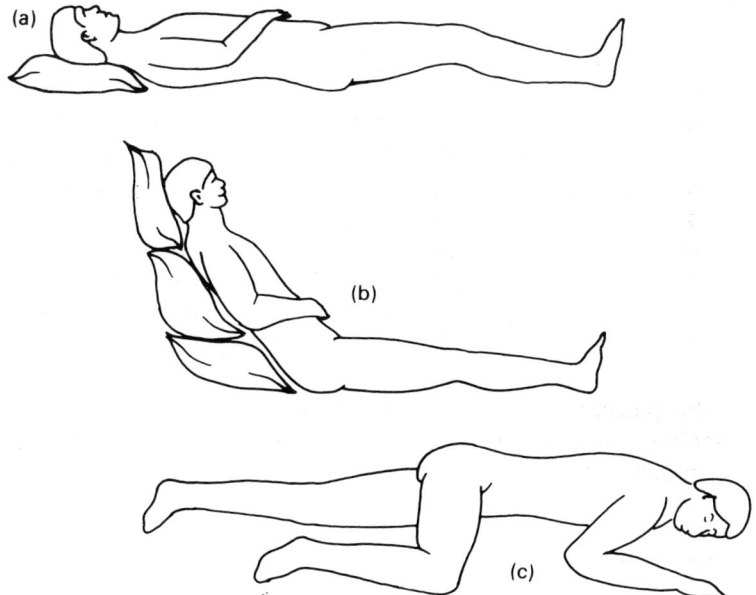

Figure 3 Diagrams of nursing positions: recumbent (a); semirecumbent (b); semiprone (c).

Once on the trolley the patient should *only* be moved when necessary:
 To be undressed.
 To be examined by the doctor.
 To prevent pressure areas — every 2 hours.
These movements must be carried out by a sufficient number of staff, with full awareness and consideration of the injuries sustained.

HEALTH AND SAFETY

Health and safety at work is now an increasing challenge. The safety precautions in the accident and emergency department are to protect all those who enter the department and all those who work in the department. Much of safety involves preventing accidents, which means being alert to potential problem areas. The main safety considerations are to ensure that the department and its equipment provide maximum protection for the patients and staff.

Department and Equipment

The Department

Although the arrangements within departments are varied there are several similarities in structure:
- Easily accessible entrance, with either a ramp or walk-way.
- Rooms or cubicles with wide entrances.
- Non slip floors.
- Easily accessible cupboards to prevent staff having to climb for articles or articles falling on staff or patients.
- Easily accessible equipment especially for emergency use.
- Patient toilet doors which have locks which open from the inside as well as the outside.

To maintain safety corridors and cubicles must not be obstructed by any unnecessary material or equipment.

The Equipment

Safe, correctly functioning equipment is essential. The equipment used is often electrical and must be checked frequently to ensure safety and accurate function.

In addition, all equipment must be used correctly to be safe. Particular caution must be taken with:
- Oxygen — may cause an explosion if used near a naked light.
- Suction apparatus — may cause or may transfer infection if the equipment used is not sterile.
- Patients' trolleys should move quietly and smoothly. Protective side rails must work on each trolley. The nurse must be able to elevate the head and foot of each trolley as necessary.

The Patient

The patient enters the department for treatment and once within the department must be protected from further injury. It is the nurses' responsibility to maintain the patient's safety.

General Guide Lines

1 Patients should be constantly observed and particular attention paid to patients who are:

Children — either the parent, the accompanying adult or the nurse should always be in attendance.

Confused — the nurse or relative, if appropiate, should stay with the patient to prevent possible self-injury through restlessness.

Violent — this patient should not be allowed to inflict injury on self or anyone else (see Chapter 12).

Acutely ill — any patient whose observations have not stabilized.

2 Regular observations should be maintained on:

Unconscious or semiconscious patients.

Epileptic patients — these patients may be drowsy but still need to be observed for possible reoccurrence of the seizure.

Patients with heart complaints.

Patients following general anaesthesia in the department.

Regular and constant observations of these patients provide immediate knowledge of a change in their condition and prevent patients from further accidental injury.

3 Explain to patients why they must remain in one place and not wander needlessly around the department; they may fall over objects, harming themselves, or obstruct staff and thereby endanger another patient.

4 Protect patients by observing the rules and regulations of drug administration. Ensure that the correct drug is being given to the correct patient.

Also before giving an antibiotic ascertain from patients whether they are allergic to antibiotics. Reaction to antibiotics can produce anaphylactic shock. (See Chapter 2).

5 Lift and move patients correctly depending on their injuries.

6 Emergency bells are situated in some departments to enable the nurse to summons assistance when patient care warrants it. To provide safe patient care the nurse must be aware of these bells, not only their operation but when they sound to provide other staff with assistance. These bells may also be used as a safety aid by nursing staff if a patient becomes violent and threatens a nurse.

The Staff

All staff within the accident and emergency department must be alert to patient safety and treatment and also self-protection.

It is essential to know how to use equipment correctly.

Lifting and moving patients improperly can cause injury to staff as well as patients. The basic principles of safer lifting must be observed:

1   Ensure that enough help is available.
2   Decide on the type of lift — *remember* this depends on the patient's injuries — and which team member will give the commands.
3   Ensure that the immediate area is clear of obstacles.
4   Ensure that the trolley's or wheelchair's brakes are on.
5   Stand with feet slightly apart.
6   Bend the knees — not the back.
7   Arrange the lift signals so that all assistants lift **together** when the elected team member gives the commands.
8   Do not attempt to lift a patient alone. Back injuries are one of the commonest injuries to nurses and once received can jeopardize and even end a career.

When dealing with a violent patient always ensure that there is adequate help or summon assistance.

Safety towards the patient involves the correct administration of nursing care.

The nurse should know the hospital procedure for various techniques in the accident and emergency department, e.g., aseptic technique; the administration of drugs.

ETHICAL AND MEDICOLEGAL ASPECTS

The ethical and medicolegal aspects of the accident and emergency department means that the treatment given must be that which is acceptable to the laws of society and that there is no negligence in the carrying out of these duties. The accident and emergency department is defined as an area which deals with any form or result of traumatic injury and any medical emergency which is threatening a person's health. This involves a tremendous range of medical knowledge.

Diagnosis and treatment are essential but diagnosis is not always easy and therefore treatment not always immediate.

Many investigations may need to be conducted to confirm a diagnosis and it is the doctor's responsibility to determine the diagnosis and commence treatment to prevent the legal litigation of neglect.
Neglect may affect the nurse if there is:
Insufficient or delayed observations.
Failure to report abnormal observations.
Delay in carrying out necessary treatments ordered.
Insufficient instructions to the patient on discharge.

Correct Treatment

1   Ensure that you are carrying out the correct treatment on the correct patient. There can often be difficulty in deciphering the doctor's written instructions — do not guess at what has been written — go and ask the doctor verbally. If drugs are to be given make sure that the doctor has clearly printed the name of the drug, the dose and route.
2   Ensure that techniques are correct, e.g., compressive bandages can be applied too tightly and result in the constriction of blood supply to the area creating further problems for the patient.
3   Ensure that an ordered drug is not administered twice by signing for it immediately it is given. In the accident and emergency department it is so easy to be diverted to other patients and although you intend to return to a certain task it is not always possible, and time does make one forget. Always sign immediately you have given a drug, also be aware of your hospital policy regarding checking and giving of drugs. Controlled drugs and insulin must be checked with a state registered nurse, all other drugs must be checked with a trained nurse, i.e., a state enrolled or state registered nurse.

CONFIDENTIALITY

Confidentiality does not mean you keep secret information for the patient. It means that the patient may talk to the nurse or doctor in private; this can often be a problem in departments with only curtains dividing some areas. Consider the patient's privacy and try not to ask questions in front of relatives, friends or other patients. The nurse must relay information provided by the patient to the doctor in order to provide complete care. Often the nurse receives information that the patient neglected to give to the doctor.

As the patient may be cared for by other nursing staff within the department any necessary information must be conveyed to the people concerned to facilitate safe patient care. This information must also be transmitted to the ward staff who care for the patient on admission to hospital.

The information conveyed in all these instances does not breach the confidentiality of the patient but is essential for patient care.

Other health personnel may be involved in the patient's care, e.g., the general practitioner or district nurse. To provide continuity of care these people are informed of the patient's attendance in the department, the care received and the patient's future needs. An example of this might be the letter the patient takes to the general practitioner following treatment for a laceration stating when the sutures are to be removed.

Confidentiality is extremely important when dealing with people not in the medical field. The nurse may come into contact with relatives or friends, the police or newspaper reporters when confidentiality has to be considered.

Relatives

When possible, relatives or friends must be informed of the patient's progress. However there may be instances when the patient does not want the relative or friend informed at all, or not informed about the actual incident or condition, e.g., the patient who has been a victim of rape; the patient who received injuries in a robbery attempt. In these instances it is the patient's wishes that must be acknowledged and adhered to.

Police

The nurse should not give evidence to the police directly. If the police require evidence from the nurse then this must be dealt with by hospital administration. This does not mean you do not speak to the police, remember they have a job to perform. Simple statements such as 'He seems to be improving' or 'The doctor is examining her at present' are quite acceptable. You may also assist the police by asking the doctor when it will be convenient for the police to interview the patient.

There are also instances when the police should be notified about a patient in the department. If you identify a patient who you know is wanted by the police, descriptions of some wanted persons are notified to the department, then discretely inform the nurse in charge of the department or the doctor so that the local police station can be notified.

Some injuries should also be notified to the police. In Britain it is illegal to have fire arms without a license, and a criminal offence to use a weapon on another person. When a patient is admitted with a bullet wound then the police, if not already involved in the case, should be notified.

Newspaper Reporters

On *no* account may a nurse give any information to reporters. The hospital administrator will deal with all public reports, and all legal matters. This also means that the nurse on duty should not be involved in signing any legal documents, e.g. a will.

PATIENTS' COMPLAINTS

Accident and emergency departments can be subjected to many complaints from patients. These vary from long waiting periods, to draughts in the department, to unsatisfactory care, and to lost articles. Each complaint must be honoured and dealt with accordingly. Many complaints may be dealt with within the department.

Long Waiting Periods

Explanations concerning the reason for long waiting periods can often prevent further complaints. It is also possible to take action to reduce long waiting periods and eliminate the problem. In some departments there are 2 or 3 doctors in attendance at one time. If for some reason only one doctor is present and the work load is excessive then the nurse should be aware of the waiting list and inform the doctor. This allows for more staff to be summoned to the department. Remember if the doctor is busy seeing patients the number of patients waiting to be seen may go unnoticed.

When the department is busy assist the doctor; this is best done by staying with the doctor as he or she examines the patient and listening to the treatment ordered. This saves the doctor having to find a nurse and repeat the treatment that has already been explained to the patient. However busy, ensure that the doctor clearly writes out the treatment.

Draughts

Alertness on the part of the nurse can prevent the problem of draughts; on cold days keep doors and windows closed. If a patient does complain of the cold ensure that there are no obvious draughts and give the patient extra blankets.

Unsatisfactory Care

Unsatisfactory care can often be a patient's complaint, however the medical notes may indicate otherwise and it is important to discover the actual complaint. It may be that the patient wanted an X-ray although the doctor did not think it necessary. Patients however insistent should not be subjected to X-rays without medical indications. Allow the patient to voice the complaint; discuss the complaint with the doctor so that you are well aware of the situation and then explain again to the patient. Your explanation may satisfy the patient as it clarifies the doctor's statements. If the patient is still not satisfied whatever the cause, senior nursing staff in the department should be consulted. The patient will be asked to make a written statement, for further action.

Lost Articles

Lost articles are a continual problem in the department. Make sure that the patient's property is always kept with the patient or in a special storage area. **Know** your hospital procedure regarding property. If a patient does complain of loss inform the senior nurse in the department. Search for the article making sure that the relatives or friends have not received it and that the patient in fact had it on admission to the department. If the article cannot be found then a written statement must be completed.

If complaints cannot be dealt with in the department then they should be stated in writing and relayed to the hospital administrator via the senior nurse in the department.

Complete and accurate documentation is essential for all nursing and medical records

The accident and emergency nurse sees and treats many patients in a day and unless treatment is clearly documented it is increasingly difficult to remember a situation which occurred several years ago and is now the subject of a legal action.

The accident and emergency nurse must be especially alert to the medicolegal aspects. By giving good, safe nursing care, many legal problems may be prevented.

REVISION OBJECTIVES

1 State the functions of the accident and emergency department.
2 Describe the role of the nurse in the department including:
   The responsibilities on the first day.
   The various examinations and investigation procedures conducted in the department and the nurse's role in relationship to the procedures.
   The treatment procedures.
   Further responsibilities to patients, relatives or friends and ward staff.
   The importance of communication.
   The challenge and uncertainty of accident and emergency work.
3 Detail the moving and lifting of patients in the department.
4 Identify basic safety precautions within the department.
5 Appreciate the ethical and medicolegal aspects of nursing within an accident and emergency department.

2
Reception and Assessment of the Patient

RECEPTION

At reception, each patient should be treated as an individual with an individual injury or illness and assessed according to individual needs. On admission to the department, the patient must be greeted and shown to an appropriate area. As the majority of patients walk into the accident and emergency department with minor complaints, the necessary information can be obtained directly from the patient or if the patient is a child from the accompanying parent or guardian.

Details about the Patient

The necessary information to obtain regarding any patient attending the department includes the immediate and prior condition, medical history and personal details.

Immediate Condition. The immediate condition will include the reason why the patient has come to the hospital and his or her actual needs. It is the most important information the nurse needs to obtain because, even if the patient has walked into the department, his or her condition might warrant immediate treatment. For example, patients who walk into the department complaining of chest pain should be treated with priority.

The initial needs of the patient are those functions compatible with life and include adequate respiratory and circulatory functions.

The nurse must appreciate the patient's immediate condition and act accordingly.

Prior Condition. The prior condition or the circumstances which have brought the patient to the hospital need to be ascertained. The patient may be conscious on admission but the reason for coming or being brought to the department may have been because of being found in an unconscious state. The situation at the time of the incident may indicate the care the patient will require. For instance, the patient who is found collapsed in a gas-filled room and receives medical treatment may also be advised to see a psychiatrist.

Medical History. The patient's previous medical history is important in that it might indicate the patient's present condition or influence the treatment. If the patient is able to give name, age and address and has been treated previously at the hospital then the medical record will show the medical history. The patient may be able to describe his or her own medical history, or identification bracelets or necklaces may indicate that there is a history of diabetes or epilepsy or that the patient is receiving drug therapy. It is especially important to be aware of the patient on anticoagulant therapy or steroid therapy.

Clerical Information. Clerical information required by the department includes the patient's name, age and address. When a patient can be identified as having attended the department previously, the medical records can be obtained.

Next of Kin or Guardian. The name and address of the patient's next of kin or guardian are needed, especially if a life-saving operation is to be carried out. In order to obtain permission (consent) for an operation the patient must be over 16 years of age and must be alert enough to understand what this consent involves. If this is not the case and the next of kin or guardian cannot be located either in person or by telephone, then the surgeon can carry out the operation with consent through one of the following:
  Two doctors who are in agreement over the urgency of surgery.
  A court order.
If the patient is aged between 16 and 18 years, the doctor may ask the patient's permission to inform the parent or guardian about any intended treatment. Permission is required from a parent or guardian for any treatment given to children under the age of 16 years.
  If children under the age of 16, unaccompanied, require urgent treatment this will be decided by the surgeon or doctor and administered as necessitated. Other cases requiring less urgent treatment may wait until the parent or guardian arrives in the

department or treatment may be carried out by verbal consent from the accompaning adult. A child must not be left unattended in the department.

ASSESSMENT ACCORDING TO PRIORITIES

Assessment of a patient in accident and emergency must be carried out in order of priority. Observations of the airway, breathing, circulation, consciousness, temperature and pain will be carried out as the condition of each patient indicates.

Airway

Is the patient's airway clear?

Breathing

With the airway clear, is the patient breathing?
1 Does the patient appear cyanosed?
2 Is the patient having difficulty in breathing — dyspnoea?
3 If the patient is breathing, are respirations normal in rate, depth and rhythm?
4 Are both sides of the chest moving together and equally?

Circulation

Is the blood circulating adequately?
1 Observe:
    Pulse rate
    Blood pressure
2 Observe any form of haemorrhage. External haemorrhage can be seen and can come from several sources:
    Arterial — bright red blood will pump out with the heart beat
    Venous — dark blood will ooze onto the skin surface
    Capillary — small amounts of blood will seep out.
Other signs which can accompany severe external haemorrhage are also indications of internal haemorrhage. The patient may appear:
    Pale and cold
    Perspiring
    Restless
    Anxious

Other indications of internal haemorrhage may include:
 Trauma showing bruising or swelling
 A distended abdomen — assessed by increasing abdominal girth measurements.
Haemorrhage reduces the circulating blood volume causing hypovolaemia.

Shock. If the reduction in circulating blood is significant the patient will present in the condition of shock. The signs of shock are:
 Pallor
 Perspiring
 Restlessness and anxiety
 Air hunger
 A low blood pressure (hypotension)
 A rapid pulse (tachycardia)

Shock is not just caused by hypovolaemia. Two other causes of shock are heart failure and a severe reaction to an allergen.
1 *Cardiogenic shock.* For some reason the heart, which serves as the pump to create a blood pressure, fails. A patient in this condition will probably complain of accompanying symptoms of chest pain or difficulty in breathing.
2 *Anaphylactic or vasodilative shock.* The patient's system violently reacts to an allergen, and the peripheral blood vessels dilate causing blood to leave the vital organs to circulate in dilated arterioles. The patient may also have an allergic rash in reaction to the foreign substance.
 Observations indicating shock **must** be notified immediately as they require urgent treatment.

Consciousness

The observation of the consciousness level is the most accurate guide to the patient's neurological condition and, like all other observations, it should be recorded every 15 minutes. It is advisable that the same nurse makes these recordings so that there is a greater constancy. First, the nurse ascertains:
 Is the patient conscious?
 If the patient is not fully alert and responsive, what is the level of consciousness?

Does the patient:
1   Respond to verbal commands accurately?
2   Move or appear to hear the verbal commands but does not respond appropriately?
3   Respond accurately to a painful stimuli, that is, does the patient knock your hand away to relieve the pain?
4   Appear to feel the pain but is not able to remove the painful stimuli?
5   Fail to respond or move at all?
Verbal commands can vary from 'Tell me your name' (to observe whether memory and speech are satisfactory) to 'Open your eyes' (to observe whether accurate movement is present).

Painful Stimuli. When there is no verbal response, painful stimuli can be applied to elicit this response. Painful stimuli can be produced by the lower part of the ear lobe being twisted or the nurse's clenched fist being rubbed firmly over the patient's sternum.

If the patient responds to the painful stimuli then the patient's nervous system has located the area of pain and caused appropriate movement.

If the patient responds to the painful stimuli but does not remove the stimuli then the nervous system can feel pain but not identify the area or cause the appropriate movement.

Pupil Reactions. Some patients may normally have dilated pupils, but it is the pupil's reaction to light that will indicate if the pupil is abnormally dilated. Patient's pupil reactions:
1   Do they constrict equally and briskly when a light is shone into the eyes?
2   What is the size of the pupils? (See Figure 4)
    Small (pinpoint)
    Normal
    Dilated (large)

A normally dilated pupil will constrict briskly when a light is shone on it, whereas an abnormally dilated pupil will constrict slowly or remain dilated.

The comparison of the size and constriction of the pupils of the eyes will indicate which side of the brain is affected. **Remember** some patients normally have unequal sized pupils. Due to these inconsistencies, pupil observations are not the most reliable

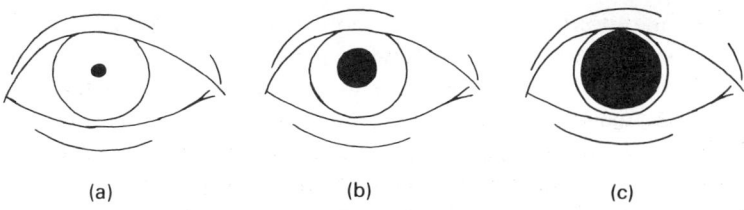

Figure 4 Pupil sizes: pinpoint (a); normal (b); dilated (c).

guide to changes in the patient's condition. However, if initial observations of a patient indicated a normal condition and subsequent observations show abnormal, these changes **must** be notified immediately.

Pupil Constriction. The constriction of the pupil of the eye is controlled by muscles in the iris. The pupil is the circular opening in the middle of the iris (also known as the 'window'). The iris is composed of two layers of muscle which lie:

Straight across the iris (Figure 5a). When these radial muscles contract the pupil becomes larger.

In a circle through the iris (Figure 5b). When these circular muscles contract then the pupil becomes smaller.

The control of these muscles is governed by the two systems of the autonomic nervous system:

The parasympathetic nervous system allows the pupil to constrict and so controls the circular muscle.

The sympathetic nervous system causes the pupil to dilate and so controls the radial muscle.

The parasympathetic and sympathetic nerve supply to the eye is carried in the *oculomotor nerves*. These are the third pair of cranial nerves and they originate from the midbrain.

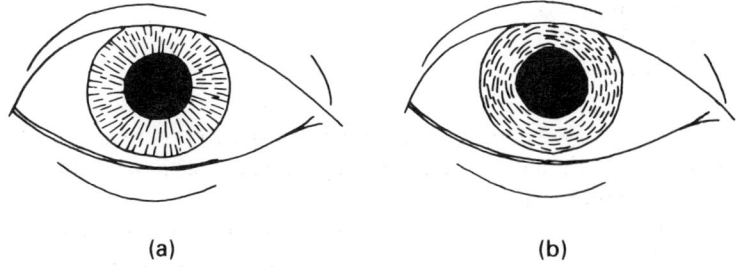

Figure 5 Muscles of the iris which allow contraction and dilation of the pupil: radial (a); circular (b).

Reason for Pupil Observation. Changes in the pupil reaction will indicate pressure on the oculomotor nerve. The pressure may be caused by swelling of brain tissue or haemorrhage within the brain. The pressure causes the brain to be displaced and forces it down to the only opening in the skull, the foramen magnum. As the oculomotor nerve runs along the base of the cerebrum from the midbrain to the eyes it is very sensitive to changes in pressure.

If the pressure is localized to one hemisphere of the brain initially then changes will appear in the pupil of the eye on that same side.

The changes that occur:
Pinpoint pupil. A pinpoint pupil means that the pupil is so constricted that it cannot get any smaller. It indicates that there is pressure on the nerve but it is still functioning. Pinpoint pupils can also indicate severe central nervous system depression as caused by an excess of opiate drugs.

Dilated fixed pupil. A dilated fixed pupil indicates severe pressure on the oculomotor nerve and the fact that the oculomotor nerve is no longer functioning. If one pupil becomes dilated and fixed, unless the pressure is relieved, this will eventually spread to the other hemisphere of the brain and affect the other eye.

Changes to notify include:
1   Deteriorating levels of consciousness.
    Voice⟶Pain⟶Nothing
2   Changes in pupil size and movement.
    Sluggish⟶Pinpoint⟶Dilated and fixed

Temperature

The body temperature, normally 37°C (98.4°F), is regulated by the nervous system. It is the hypothalamus in the brain which is sensitive to temperature changes. Temperature changes are registered in two ways:
 By the temperature of the blood passing through the hypothalamus.
 Messages from nerve endings in the skin which are stimulated by hot or cold.

Routes. The nurse after choosing the appropriate thermometer may use one of the following routes:
   Oral for 1 minute
   Axilla or groin for 5 minutes
   Rectal for 1 minute

The most accurate recording of body temperature is by rectum and this method is used on:
   Babies and young children
   Patients with noticeable changes in body temperature, e.g., a high temperature *(pyrexia)* or a low temperature *(hypothermia)*. With hypothermia, the patient will be cold to touch and appear pale or blue in colour. With pyrexia, the patient will be warm, perspiring and flushed in appearance.
Normal thermometers only record temperatures down to 35°C. If a patient's temperature is unrecordable on a normal thermometer then a subnormal thermometer must be used rectally. These thermometers record temperatures as low as 32°C.

Changes. Changes in temperature recordings can result from:
   Damage to the hypothalamus — usually in cases of head injury.
   Prolonged exposure to cold temperatures — usually aggravated by inactivity.
   Bacterial infection within the body.

Pain

One of the commonest complaints which brings a patient to the accident and emergency department is pain. It can often be diagnostic of the patient's condition. Pain is registered and brought to the consciousness of the patient by the nervous system. It is said that pain is a protective defence mechanism of the body, as it indicates that something is wrong and the cause needs correction. Pain may also act as a deterrent to further damage as it may stop a patient from moving and creating additional problems, e.g., fractures.

Causes. Pain is caused by:
1 A protective mechanism of the peripheral nervous system which records hot and cold, thereby preventing burns or frostbite.
2 Irritation. Nerve endings may be abnormally stimulated by foreign or harmful substances such as chemicals or bacteria.
3 Abnormal muscular activity, especially increased muscle activity of smooth, involuntary muscle, e.g., the muscles that produce peristalsis.
4 Disturbance in the blood supply to the tissues causes hypoxia and results in the build up of waste products. This occurs in ischaemia and may lead to tissue death (*necrosis*). Pain following strenuous exercise is due to an accumulation of a waste product, lactic acid, and generally takes several days before it can be removed from the body.

Systemic Changes. Pain may produce systemic changes:
   Increased blood pressure
   Increased pulse
   Increased respirations
   Dilated pupils
   Perspiration
These effects are being produced by the sympathetic nervous system as it responds to the stress situation of the body.

Location. The location or sites of pain can be related to anatomical structures, e.g., chest to heart; right epigastric region to gall bladder; right iliac fossa (McBurney's point) to appendix.
With children it is often difficult to distinguish the cause of the pain. Children must be observed to see if they hold or rub a particular area of their body, e.g., an ear, in an attempt to relieve pain. The history from the parent or guardian is essential to ascertain the cause.

Radiation. Pain can radiate away from the site of the causative factor due to the nerve distribution of the body and can be recorded elsewhere, e.g.,
   Heart — pain may move down left arm or up into left side of jaw
   Gall-bladder — pain may be located between the shoulder blades

Appendix — inflammation of the appendix may present initially with generalized abdominal pain or midepigastric pain

Type. The type or character of pain can be hard to describe as pain can manifest itself in so many ways, from mild to severe. The severity of pain is difficult to judge as patients have their own responses which are often based on cultural patterns. Some patients try to bear pain quietly whereas others feel that pain is relieved by verbal expression. The nurse's attitude should be one that encourages and allows the patient to explain the sort of pain felt, without putting words into the patient's mouth. While the patient is describing the pain, observe any movements as this can be very indicative and aid diagnosis, e.g.,
  Pointing to a spot with a finger means that the pain is well localized.
  Fingers outspread across the abdomen means a vacillating pain.
A **burning** pain feels hot and is often associated with irritation or inflammation. The patient with gastritis will complain of a hot, burning feeling in the midepigastric region.
Severe intractable pain is associated with the obstruction of blood to the tissues *(ischaemia)*. Partial obstruction such as angina or intermittent claudication results in a severe pain which is relieved by rest which allows blood to return to the tissues. Complete obstruction such as a myocardial infarction results in continuous pain. The pain is gripping and crushing.
Intermittent pain is associated with involuntary muscular action. The pain increases on muscular contraction and is known as a spasmodic colic pain. This is associated with obstructions in areas of involuntary muscle, such as the gastrointestinal tract and urinary tract.

Duration. The nurse must determine how long the pain has been present; whether it is acute or chronic; whether anything can relieve it; and whether anything particularly aggravates it, e.g.,
  The pain of a traumatic incident will be immediate.
  Irritating pain such as gastritis may be relieved by food particularly bland food. Food will coat the stomach and prevent the hydrochloric acid burning the irritated stomach lining.

Eating fatty foods may aggravate the pain of a gall-bladder condition.

Other Problems. Be observant for other problems which may accompany pain:
Nausea and vomiting
Faintness
Muscle spasm or rigidity

General Observations

General observations of a patient mean the nurse must:
Listen. Listen to the patient and take note of this in relation to the patient's condition. The patient may complain of:
Tenderness
Pain
Loss of sensation
Loss of movement

Look. Look at the patient and observe:
Obvious injury:
Bruising
Laceration
Swelling
Deformity
Lack of movement
Broken or ulcerated skin
Skin appearance:
Loss of normal colour, ashen or putty coloured, generally pallid
Cyanosed
Jaundiced

When a patient is jaundiced in appearance there may be additional problems if there is bleeding due to a clotting defect. The patient might require vitamin K administration.

Touch. Touch the patient's skin. The state of the skin can indicate the possible condition of the patient and previous mental or physical state of health, i.e., has the patient neglected his or her general health both in nutrition and hygiene. The skin may be:

Dry
Moist
Cold
Warm

There may be a rash present.

Detect Odour. A particular odour may indicate the cause of, or be the result of, the patient's condition.

Indicates the cause
  Alcohol
  Acetone
Result of condition
  Vomit
  Incontinence

The nurse's assessment of the patient in the accident and emergency department is vital, and the nurse demonstrates the importance through accuracy in observation, recording and reporting. The patient's condition **must** be assessed and appropriate treatment commenced, with life-sustaining procedures carried out **immediately**.

PATIENT CARE

On admission to the department the patient must be greeted and shown to an appropriate area.

Positioning

The nurse must decide on a suitable position for a patient. Many patients can be treated while sitting in a chair. However, the nurse must assess each patient to determine the correct position:
A breathless patient will need to sit up, usually on a trolley and be well supported with a back rest, pillows and cot sides.
A patient with a back injury will need to lie flat on his or her back (recumbent).
A patient in the condition of shock, will need to be placed in a recumbent position, that is, flat with one pillow or with the foot of the trolley elevated so that the head is lower.
Exceptions to this are:
1 The patient who has had a myocardial infarction (see Chapter 5) but is breathless. This patient may need to be in a semi-recumbent position to aid breathing although suffering from hypotension, tachycardia and signs of shock.

2 The patient who has an acute abdomen from a perforation (see Chapter 9). This patient may have all the signs of shock but, if the blood pressure is **NOT** decreased, will need to be kept semirecumbent to prevent the gastrointestinal contents from touching the diaphragm and causing possible respiratory or liver problems.

The patient who has severe internal or external bleeding from a limb. Due to the condition of shock the patient can be nursed in a recumbent position but the affected limb can be elevated in an attempt to stop the bleeding.

The patient with a fracture. The position of the patient will depend on the bone that is fractured. Whatever the position the fractured bone or bones must be kept immobilized. Special care must be taken when undressing these patients.

Children if placed on stretchers should have the safety rails up in position and always be accompanied by an adult. Alternatively, depending on the condition, the child may sit on the parent's or guardian's lap and be held securely.

Preparation for Examination

The positioning and preparation of the patient for examination is the nurse's responsibility. The nurse must prepare the patient for the doctor's examination. The patient will be undressed appropriately and put in a hospital gown.

While undressing the patient, the nurse is able to observe the state and appearance of the patient's skin. During this stage, however, it is vital that the nurse is aware of the patient's condition and the nature of the injuries to know how best to remove the patient's clothing. If a patient's clothing has to be cut off, when possible, cut along the seams.

PATIENT'S BELONGINGS

Clothing

Any clothing which is removed from the patient should be stored in an appropriate place. If the patient is on a trolley clothing is put in the container on the bottom or placed by the patient if the patient is sitting on a chair.

Some departments record all clothing and valuables which patients bring with them. Take especial care of:

Dentures. If dentures are removed from a patient's mouth, and it is essential that they are if the patient is unconscious, the nurse must ensure that they are put with the patient's property in a labelled container.

Spectacles. Spectacles are placed **safely** in with the patient's property. Some departments may put spectacles in with valuables and keep them in the hospital safe.

Contact Lenses. Patients should wear their contact lenses **only** if they can open and close their eyes normally. Any disturbance in conscious level or injury in the vicinity of the eyes should require that these lenses are removed. If the lenses are removed they must be stored appropriately to prevent complications and damage to them. Containers should be marked 'left' and 'right' and the corresponding lenses put in each container. Soft contact lenses require storage in a solution so that they do not dry out. If the patient does not have the solution to hand sterile water may be used.

Valuables

Some departments require that all valuables belonging to a patient are listed and stored in the hospital safe until the patient is discharged or requests them.

Other departments require the recording and storage of valuables only for those patients who are confused, unconscious or who state that they would like their valuables put in the safe. Sometimes a patient's watch is removed quickly to erect an intravenous infusion; remember that it is a valuable item.

Elderly patients may state that they have only a little money on them but the amount should be verified. It has been known for this to be said when, in fact, the patient has been found to have £1000. Large sums of money must be put in the hospital safe to prevent loss.

Patients who refuse to put valuables in the hospital safe are to be advised that they keep the valuables at their own risk. Some departments may require these patients to sign a form declaring that they are keeping their valuables with them.

With children it is important to allow them to keep a toy, such as a teddy bear, as this provides them with some security and familiarity. It may even be necessary to use the teddy bear as a patient and clean its foot and apply a plaster to obtain a child's co-operation. Many departments now keep a supply of toys so that, if a child has come without a toy, one can be provided.

RELATIVES

When a seriously ill patient is brought into the department, there is seldom time to deal with relatives or the accompanying friend. Even so, it is important to help those accompanying the patient at this time. A quick word from the nurse can help both the relative or friend and the patient. The more information that can be obtained about the patient and his or her condition the more accurately treatment can be commenced.

A child or children accompanying the ill patient must not be left unattended in the department. Voluntary workers, the receptionist or a nurse, if available, may look after these children. It is essential that they are taken care of and that the nurse attends to this.

The Role of the Nurse

Role of the nurse with relatives or friends:
1   Ask them to go to the receptionist and give all relevant information about the patient if necessary.
2   Allow them to sit in the waiting area or in a quiet room when possible while the patient is being treated. If there is available staff then it is comforting to offer a cup of tea.
3   Make sure that they are informed of the patient's condition. Initial resuscitative procedures on a patient may take up to 30 minutes. Whilst for the busy nurse the time passes amazingly quickly, for the waiting relatives or friends each minute can seem an hour and to them 'no news' does not necessarily mean 'good news'. Ensure that they are informed of the patient's condition as soon as possible. Simple statements such as 'The doctor is examining the patient at present' at least indicates that the patient is still alive. Whether the patient will survive is a constant worry for those accompanying the patient and they will not be convinced until they have seen the patient themselves. Allow them to see the patient as soon as it is possible.
4   When relatives or friends must be told that the patient's

condition has deteriorated since coming into the department this may create problems. Whenever possible the relatives or friends should be seated in a quiet room and made comfortable and told by the doctor or by the nurse in charge.

Death

On the death of a patient, the relatives or friends should be allowed some time to assimilate the fact of death. The nurse must then decide whether to stay during this period or allow the relatives or anyone else accompanying the patient, a short time alone. Again, a cup of tea often helps during this period.

They must also be allowed to see the patient if they so wish. Before taking the relatives or friends to the patient, ensure that the patient is clean and peaceful and placed in a single room. Always escort the relatives or friends and make sure that there are chairs beside the patient. Stay in the room until they leave. Be ready to answer any questions.

Make sure that the spiritual needs of the patient have been met, or are met; this may involve the services of:

A priest to administer the last offices if the patient is a Catholic.

A rabbi or family member to recite psalms for a Jewish patient.
   Last offices can be conducted by a rabbi or family member, or nurses wearing disposable gloves so as not to defile the body.

A family member or Muslim to recite verses from the Koran for a Muslim patient. On death, the patient's head must be turned towards the right shoulder so the patient can be buried facing Mecca. The last offices are conducted by a Muslim of the same sex or by the nursing staff wearing disposable gloves.

The eldest son of a male member of the Hindu religion for a Hindu patient. There is no ritual washing of the body after death so last offices can be carried out by the nursing staff.

Before the relatives or friends leave, make sure that they are well enough to go home. If alone make arrangements that he or she is accompanied if possible. Grief can bring about a variety of actions in a person including a change in physical or psychological health.

General Advice

Relatives or friends can create problems in small overcrowded departments and may hinder the care of the patient so to avoid this problem, when possible, advise the relative or friend to:

1   Stay with the patient and not move unnecessarily around the department. In some cases the person may be helping in the care of the patient, especially if it is a child or a confused, restless patient. If a relative or friend is there to stay with the patient to prevent further injury, the person must realize the importance of not moving from the patient's area without informing a member of the nursing staff. However, do not leave the relative unattended for long periods but return at least every 15 minutes to observe the patient and reassure the relative or friend.

2   Have only one member of the family present or one friend with the patient. It is impossible for busy nursing staff to answer questions to individual members of the family or friend, so it is advisable to have one person responsible for receiving information regarding the patient's condition, but make sure that you keep this member informed.

3   Patients should not be given food or drink in the accident and emergency department without the permission of the doctor. Ensure that waiting relatives or friends are informed as to whether a patient may have a drink or not.

Relatives or friends can often help the patient and generally are only too willing to do so. In a busy department, it is easier for a relative or friend to go for a cup of tea for the patient, if allowed, than for the patient to be left waiting without food or drink, because the nursing staff are otherwise engaged.

4   If the patient has been positioned in a certain way due to the injury sustained, alert the attending relative or friend as to why the patient is **not** to be moved or repositioned. For example, a patient with a back injury may be in a recumbent position although still suffering pain and a relative may attempt to alleviate the discomfort by changing the patient's position.

REVISION OBJECTIVES

1 List the information that is required from each patient on admission to the accident and emergency department.
2 Describe the assessment of a patient according to priorities.
3 Identify the condition of shock.
4 Describe and explain the significance of neurological observations.
5 Consider the effects and character of pain experienced by patients.
6 List the general observations of a patient.
7 Describe the care of a patient on admission to the department.
8 Outline the care of the relatives or friends within the department.

3
Emergency Assessment and Management

CLEAR AIRWAY

Patients who require assistance to maintain a clear airway will have some form of upper airway obstruction and may be unconscious. The obstruction can be caused by:
Foreign bodies
The tongue
Swelling of the upper respiratory tract
Trauma to the upper airway

Maintaining a Clear Airway

Loosen any tight clothing around the neck and upper chest. Remove any possible causes of obstruction.

Dentures

Foreign Bodies. Foreign bodies such as coins or nuts may be removed by inserting a finger into the mouth and removing the object.

Undigested Food or Vomitus. Undigested food or vomitus can be removed manually with the finger or by using suction apparatus. If the obstructing food bolus is further along the alimentary tract and it is impossible to remove it manually, then removal of food obstructing the airway can be achieved by using the Heimlich manoeuvre. This is generally a first aid measure and is used on a conscious patient who appears to be choking. The manoeuvre consists of:
1   Striking the patient on the back between the shoulder blades 4 times.
2   Standing behind the patient, and with both arms encircling his or her waist, allowing the patient to bend slightly forward.

Then, clenching one hand into a fist and placing it over the epigastric area of the patient's abdomen, place your other hand over your clenched fist and suddenly and forcefully compress the patient's abdomen in an upward direction. This vigorous compression which may be repeated several times should force the patient's diaphragm upwards causing pressure on the lungs, thereby creating an increased intrathoracic pressure which will in turn produce a forced expiration. The pressure of the forced expiration should remove the obstructing food bolus.

The Heimlich manoeuvre can also be carried out with the patient in a recumbent position. This time you stand by the side of the patient and compress the abdomen from the front.

Tongue. If the patient has lost the reflex actions of coughing and swallowing, or is unable to control the tongue's movement, the tongue may fall backwards and obstruct the airway. These reflex actions of coughing and swallowing are controlled by the medulla oblongata in the brain stem.

Several methods may be used to prevent the tongue from obstructing the airway:

1 Positioning the patient's head straight and moving the jaw upwards and outwards by placing your thumbs or fingers against the jaw bone (mandible) beneath the ear of the patient and pushing the jaw forward (Figure 6).

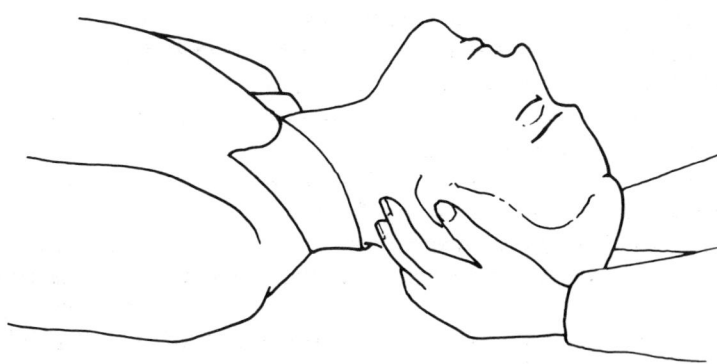

Figure 6 Maintaining the airway with little movement of the patient; hands positioned on either side of the head, with fingers pushing the jaw upwards and forwards.

Emergency Assessment & Management

2   By placing the patient in a semiprone position. *Check* before the patient is moved that the moves necessary to place him or her in a semiprone position are planned so that there is no risk of the patient's injuries being aggravated.
3   Placing an artificial airway in the patient's mouth.

Intubation

If these methods are unsuccessful in maintaining a clear airway then the patient may require intubation with either an endotracheal tube or a tracheostomy tube.

Endotracheal Tube. The passing of an endotracheal tube (intubation) is carried out by trained personnel so the anaesthetist must be contacted. The nurse can prepare the equipment the anaesthetist will require:
   Laryngoscope. This instrument should be checked daily to ensure that both the battery and the bulb are in correct working order.
   Endotracheal tube. As these tubes come in various sizes the nurse should have a selection of tubes ready and ask the anaesthetist which one is required.
   Lubricating jelly, if used.
   20 ml syringe
   One pair of Spencer Wells forceps
   Tape to tie the tube in place. Also have available an Ambu bag with a mask and an appropriate sized connection to adapt the Ambu bag to the required endotracheal tube.
Ensure the availability of:
   Oxygen
   Suction equipment

Tracheostomy Tube. Inserting a tracheostomy tube involves a surgical procedure and each department should have a sterile pack of the appropriate instruments to perform the operation. When time and conditions permit the procedure should be performed in an operating theatre, but this can often be performed within the accident and emergency department. If this is the case ensure that the room is prepared and add to the equipment the appropriate size and type of tracheostomy tube.

BREATHING

Once the airway has been cleared it must be ascertained that the patient is breathing by observing or feeling the chest for movement or testing for air movement at the nostrils.

Chest Movement. Observing the chest for movement: clothing must be removed from the chest to allow observation. Concern over the patient's respiratory function does not allow time to undress the patient completely but clothing must be removed from the chest.
  Feeling the chest for movement: if chest movement is not obvious the patient may still be breathing but the breathing may be very shallow. To check further you can place your hand flat on the patient's chest in order to feel if there is movement.

Air Movement. The palm of the hand placed lightly over the patient's nostrils will also test for the movement of air as the patient exhales.

Resuscitation

If there are no signs of respiration make sure that the patient's airway is not obstructed (see p.38) and then start the resuscitation procedure. Various hospitals have different resuscitation procedures, so you must know the procedure followed in the hospital in which you are working.
  One general resuscitation procedure would be:
1 With the patient in the recumbent position extend neck by placing one hand behind the neck of the patient and one on the patient's forehead.
2 Move thumb and forefinger of the hand on the patient's forehead over the patient's nose and pinch the nostrils together.
3 Take a deep breath in and then place your mouth over the patient's mouth and breath out gently one normal breath.
4 Observe the patient's chest to see if the air is entering the chest. Mouth-to-mouth resuscitation is not advisable in all cases especially when the patient is known to have an infection such as tuberculosis of the lung. In this case and, where available, a Brook's airway should be used or a correctly fitting mask with an Ambu bag. Two quick ventilations of the patient's lungs must be carried out initially.

Help **must** be summoned so be sure you know the appropriate call statement for your hospital.

Circulatory Function

Observation must be made of the patient's circulatory function. A patient may have a heart beat for a period of approximately three minutes even though there is no respiratory function. Check the circulatory function by placing the index and second finger together on one side of the larynx and the thumb on the other to feel the carotid pulse. If the carotid pulse cannot be felt cardiac massage must be started to maintain the patient's circulation. If the carotid pulse is present but respiratory function still absent, the ventilation of the patient's lungs must be continued at a rate of 20-24 times a minute. The normal respiratory rate is 16 times a minute.

During each respiration a person breathes in air containing:
  Oxygen 20 %
  Carbon dioxide 0.04 %
  Nitrogen 79 %

This is not the composition of air that a patient receives while being ventilated by mouth-to-mouth resuscitation. The patient receives expired air which contains:
  Oxygen 16 %
  Carbon dioxide 4 %
  Nitrogen 79 %

The difference in the vital oxygen the patient requires is 4 % less than normal and this is why respiratory resuscitation is carried out at an increased rate to normal respiration.

When the Ambu bag is used this can be connected directly to an oxygen supply to provide the patient with sufficient oxygen. However, the mask of the Ambu bag must fit securely around the patient's nose and mouth or both the pressure and the oxygen content of air entering the lungs are decreased. If the patient is unable to ventilate his or her lungs adequately then this function will be maintained by mechanical ventilation.

Mechanical Ventilation

For the patient to have mechanical ventilation either an endotracheal tube or a tracheostomy tube must be used. The anaesthetist will insert the endotracheal tube as, in Britain, this is not yet a responsibility of nursing staff or ambulance personnel. Surgery as previously mentioned is necessary to insert a tracheostomy tube.

The decision for mechanical ventilation is reached when there is an absence of respiratory function or inadequate exchange of gases in the lungs. This is determined by blood gas estimations of oxygen and carbon dioxide content.

Blood Gas Estimations

Blood for blood gas estimations is taken from the femoral or from the radial artery and must be taken into a syringe containing heparin to prevent the blood from coagulating. The blood must be kept cool to prevent changes that will alter the recordings of oxygen and carbon dioxide.

If the doctor wants to take blood for blood gases the nurse must prepare:

Syringe (2 ml) and needle (intramuscular)
Heparin
Cup with ice if available

The nurse must notify the hospital porter or transporter to take the blood to the laboratory immediately. Some departments may have the blood gas analyser in the department and will be able to conduct their own test.

Patient Care. Care of a patient who is giving blood for blood gas estimations involves:

1 When possible, the procedure must be explained to the patient.
2 The patient must be gently restrained to prevent the needle being removed while blood is being aspirated.
3 Following the removal of the blood the puncture site of the needle must be compressed firmly for a period of five minutes. This is essential as an artery has been opened by the needle and bleeding will occur until the blood-clotting mechanism is complete. Compressing prevents bleeding.

Respiratory Observations

When the patient is breathing, the nurse must determine whether respirations are satisfactory. This can be determined by observing the chest movement, the rate of respirations, signs of inadequate oxygen exchange and difficulty in breathing.

Chest Movement. Observe the chest movement and especially observe for part of the chest wall moving in opposition to the rest of the thoracic cavity *(flail chest)*. If part of the chest wall is moving in opposition it must be supported to help to maintain the correct pressures within the chest for inspiration and expiration. Place a firm bandage around the patient's chest and turn the patient towards the injured side to provide support. Before moving a patient check for possible other injuries to be sure that movement does not aggravate injuries.

Rate of Respirations. Observe the rate of respirations. Rapid respirations mean that the patient is *hyperventilating*, exhaling increased amounts of carbon dioxide, which can lead to electrolyte disturbances (see p.47). A decreased respiratory rate, *hypoventilating*, is generally due to a disorder of the central nervous system. This condition can be induced by an excess of narcotic drugs, e.g., morphine, (see Chapter 8).

Signs of Inadequate Oxygen Exchange. Observe the patient for signs of inadequate oxygen exchange. Observe the patient for signs of *hypoxia*, a diminished amount of oxygen to the tissues. Hypoxia will manifest itself as cerebral disturbance or cyanosis. The treatment is the administration of oxygen which must be given with caution.

The respiratory stimulus is believed to be governed by the amount of carbon dioxide in the blood. Patients who have chronic lung disease have a higher percentage of carbon dioxide in the blood than normal, therefore their respiratory centre is stimulated by a higher level of carbon dioxide. To replace carbon dioxide suddenly with administered oxygen may disturb the respiratory stimulus in these patients. This means that the rate of oxygen the patient is receiving is now monitored. The nurse must be sure to know the exact amount of oxygen the patient should receive.

Air contains 20 % oxygen and a Ventimask can give varying concentrations of oxygen, e.g., 24 %, 28 %, 35 %, and 38 %. A MC mask can supply oxygen at the rate of 2 litres per minute giving 36.8 % oxygen.

All oxygen administered should be humidified as oxygen dries mucous membranes and the dryness can cause irritation.

Giving excess oxygen to a patient will decrease the respiratory rate and make a patient become restless. The patient's skin may become bright pink in appearance. The adminstration of oxygen in this case must be decreased or discontinued.

Precautions with Oxygen

Oxygen aids combustion. Make sure that no one smokes in the vicinity of the oxygen being used and make sure that no electrical or mechanical equipment is used nearby as they may generate sparks.

Ensure that when the patient is moved and requires oxygen that the oxygen cylinder on the trolley is sufficiently full and is connected to the patient.

Difficulty in Breathing. Observe the patient for signs of difficulty in breathing *(dyspnoea)*. Difficulty may be due to an obstructed airway, if so this should be cleared (see p. 38). Pain in the thoracic region may limit chest expansion causing both dyspnoea and inadequate oxygen exchange. Analgesia may be administered. (See Chapter 6 for further details).

CIRCULATION

It must be ascertained that the patient's blood circulation is adequate. Immediate observations of the carotid pulse (see p. 42) will reveal whether the patient requires cardiac resuscitation. If so, **commence** immediately.

Cardiac Arrest

Before working in an accident and emergency department, nursing staff should be familiar with the cardiac techniques and procedures of the department and know who and what number to call. The accident and emergency department of a hospital is often the safest place in which to require resuscitation because there are usually several trained people present initially. The department might even have been alerted to the arrival of a patient who has a cardiac arrest, by telephone from ambulance control, in which case the following will have been prepared:

The area and trolley
The anaesthetist's equipment
Oxygen
Suction
Defibrillator and cardiac monitor

An intravenous infusion with sodium bicarbonate

A cut down set. This is a sterile pack to enable the doctor to incise the patient's skin and reach a deep vein to commence an intravenous infusion.

Drugs, syringes and needles (intramuscular, intrathoracic and intravenous)

The members of the cardiac arrest team, the doctor, the anaesthetist and the nursing officer, will also be present.

Cardiac Resuscitation

The most important factor is that the nurse recognizes the need for resuscitation and then acts accordingly and calls for help. Cardiac resuscitation is compressing the heart in an attempt to circulate blood around the body. To compress the heart sufficiently the rib cage must be depressed at least 3-4 cm. It is important to apply pressure to the correct area of the chest. To find the correct area:

1   Locate the Xiphoid process — the small triangle of cartilage at the lower end of the sternum — and place 2 fingers over this.
2   Rest the heel of your other hand on the sternum and against your 2 fingers so that the heel of your hand is in the correct position.
3   Bring your locating hand and place it on top of the hand on the sternum.
4   Apply pressure evenly and smoothly. Keep your elbows straight as this allows the application of more pressure. Your hands should be kept on the patient's chest.

Moving your hands off the chest between compression can create two main problems:

Incorrect positioning when hands are replaced for the next compression.

Incorrect direction of force which may result in fracturing of ribs.

The compressions squeeze the heart between the sternum and the vertebrae and create the pressure to pump blood. Once the heart has been compressed it will take time for blood to re-enter the heart. In normal health the heart refills approximately 72 times a minute. When you massage a patient's heart, it is not as efficient so the rate is a little faster, approximately 100 times a minute. Most hospitals resuscitate a patient using a ratio of 1:5, i.e., one ventilation to five cardiac compressions. This means that if the heart is compressed 100 times per minute then the patient is also ventilated at the rate of 20 times per minute. If two people perform this procedure they **must** work to the same ratio because a patient's lungs cannot be ventilated when the sternum is compressed. It is advisable for the person performing the cardiac massage to count the compressions and then allow the ventilation. Timing of the speed of compression can best be achieved by counting aloud in thousands: One thousand — two thousand — three thousand — four thousand — five thousand and compressing the sternum on each number.

Functions in Resuscitation

The most important functions in resuscitation are to:
1 Ventilate the lungs — oxygen must be supplied to be circulated to the tissues.
2 Maintain heart function — the heart function should be monitored on a cardiac monitor. To do this the electrodes must be connected to the patient and the machines switched on (see Chapter 5).
3 Correct the changes which are occurring within the body. Due to the lack of or deficient circulation within the body oxygen is unable to get to the tissues and waste products are unable to be removed from the body. This results in the electrolyte balance of the body being disturbed producing a *metabolic acidosis*. An increase in acid (waste products) within the body usually stimulates the respiratory centre and respirations are increased so that carbon dioxide is expelled in an attempt to correct the imbalance. In the case of a cardiac arrest there is no respiratory function so the imbalance must be corrected from an acid towards an alkaline level. This is done by administering sodium bicarbonate (8.4 %) intravenously and should be **commenced** at once. The intravenous infusion must be administered as soon as possible because as the blood stops circulating the veins, due to their thin muscular walls, collapse. Collapsed veins create difficulty for the doctor trying to locate a suitable vein to commence the infusion. The nurse can assist by placing a tourniquet around the patient's limb and possibly putting the limb in a dependent position in an attempt to dilate a vein. If the doctor is unable to locate a superficial vein then the equipment must be set up for a cut down to a deep vein (see p. 46).

Heart Action after Cardiac Arrest

The patient who has a cardiac arrest will have a tracing on the cardiac monitor of either: cardiac asystole or ventricular fibrillation.

Cardiac asystole means that there is no heart action and treatment to stimulate heart action includes:

Adrenaline 1:1000 which increases the strength of ventricular contractions and produces vasoconstriction. Adrenaline can be administered directly into the heart muscle using a cardiac needle. Following its administration cardiac massage is continued and the monitor is observed for the return of the patient's heart action.

Ventricular fibrillation means the heart muscle is quivering but not beating with enough force or purpose to circulate the blood. Treatment to produce effective heart action includes:

The use of the defibrillator with which the patient receives an electrical shock of approximately 200 J.

Drugs: Use and Action

Drugs which may be given to a patient during cardiac arrest vary depending on the actual heart action. During a cardiac arrest drugs can be given in quick succession. It is important that the nurse records the type of drugs given, the amount and the time.

Decreased Heart Rate. For a decreased heart rate, drugs which can be administered include:

Atropine sulphate 0.3 - 0.6 mg increases the heart rate. It is given intramuscularly or intravenously.

Dopamine hydrochloride (Intropin) 200 mg increases the blood pressure. It is given intravenously.

Isoprenaline (Saventrine) is a cardiac stimulant. It is usually given intravenously in 1 litre of dextrose.

Calcium chloride 1.7 - 3.4 mmol dose. Calcium in a correct amount is essential for cardiac muscle to function. It is given intravenously.

Irregular Heart Action. For an irregular heart action, drugs which can be administered include:

Lignocaine hydrochloride 50 - 100 mg. It is given intravenously.

Practolol (Eraldin) 5 - 25 mg. It treats atrial and ventricular arrhythmias and is given intravenously.

Procainamide hydrochloride (Pronestyl). This decreases the excitability of the heart muscle and so slows down and regulates the conduction of nerve impulses through the heart. It is given intravenously.

Increased Heart Action. For an increased heart action, digoxin can be administered:.

Digoxin (Lanoxin) slows, steadies and strengthens the heart action. It can be given intravenously or intramuscularly.

Respiratory Problems. For respiratory problems, drugs which can be given include:

Aminophylline (Cardophyline) 250 mg. It relaxes the bronchial muscle and relieves pulmonary oedema. It is given intravenously.

Salbutamol (Ventolin) is given intravenously, intramuscularly or orally.

Other Drugs. Other drugs which can be given include:

Frusemide (Lasix) 20 - 80 mg is a diuretic. It can be given intravenously or intramuscularly.

Calcium chloride 1.7 - 3.4 mmol increases the tone of cardiac muscle. It can be given intravenously or intramuscularly.

Diazepam (Valium) reduces the incidence of ectopic beats.

Hydrocortisone is an anti-inflammatory drug. It also allows the body to react to a stressful situation by accentuating the action of the adrenal glands.

Outcome of Resuscitation

Successful resuscitation results in the return of an adequate circulatory function. The patient must then be admitted to hospital for further observation and treatment.

If the patient arrived in the department with a relative or friend, the nurse must inform the concerned party as soon as possible regarding the patient's condition.

In the event of death in the department, the nurse must:
Ensure that the doctor has certified that the patient is dead.
Remove the body to a suitable area where it can be made presentable.

Remember that:
1 The relatives may wish to see the body.
2 Sudden death requires a coroner's inquiry, and if the deceased must undergo a postmortem to confirm the cause of death, this may mean that the body is **not** to be disturbed. Ascertain the policy of your hospital concerning Last Offices. The patient must be identified and when possible this is done within the department or by the next of kin when located. If the patient is unknown then the body must have an identifying label. Clothing and valuables must be recorded and made available for the next of kin to collect.

Changes in Circulatory Function

Accurate and frequent observations **must** be made (every 15 minutes initially) of the changes in the circulatory function of the seriously ill patient. To assess changes in the function of the circulatory system blood pressure and pulse are recorded.

Blood Pressure

The normal blood pressure recording is 120 systolic over 70 diastolic.

Changes to Notify. Changes to notify include a fall in blood pressure *(hypotension)* which may only be recordable by feeling the radial pulse palpation. If the blood pressure is 90 systolic or below, the doctor should be notified. Severe hypotension indicates the condition of shock and requires treatment (see p.51).

A rise in blood pressure *(hypertension)*, when the blood pressure may be 200 systolic over 110 diastolic, is also notifiable. Hypertension increases the pressure within arteries and may cause weakness of the arterial walls and also means the heart is under pressure when it is at rest *(diastolic)* The blood pressure **must** be decreased. In the case of a patient who is unconscious an increasing blood pressure will indicate increasing intracranial pressure which **must** be relieved.

The Pulse

The pulse rate will alter in accordance with the blood pressure. This will indicate hypotension, resulting in an increased heart rate, *tachycardia*, which is a sign of shock and an increased attempt to circulate blood around the body; or, hypertension, resulting in a decreased heart rate, *bradycardia*, in order for the heart to beat with more force.

The alteration in pulse rhythm and volume can also result from heart conditions.

Haemorrhage and Shock

Haemorrhage **must** be recognized as severe haemorrhage produces the condition of shock. External haemorrhage can be seen but internal haemorrhage must be determined.

Internal

Internal haemorrhage, or bleeding, can be suspected from the following observations:
- Patient is pale, cold, perspiring, restless, anxious and even confused.
- Tachycardia
- Hypotension
- Breathlessness
- Possible swelling related to site of trauma, e.g., around fracture of femur

Internal bleeding can manifest itself in:
- *Haemoptysis* — coughing blood
- *Haematemesis* — vomiting blood
- *Malaena* — black, tarry faeces which indicate bleeding in the gastrointestinal tract as the blood has undergone changes as it passes along the gastrointestinal tract.
- *Haematuria* — blood in the urine

If the internal bleeding is sufficient the patient will be in a condition of shock and will require immediate treatment for this condition.

Patient Care

Blood is an extremely distressing sight for patients, especially if it is their own, so that reassurance and prompt treatment are essential.

In the case of haemoptysis it is important to maintain the patient's airway. Ensure that the patient has a vomit bowl and that suction equipment is available for use. When the patient's condition is stable a mouthwash should be given.

If a patient has haematemesis the same treatment is required as for haemoptysis. In addition to this, it is important to prevent inhalation of the vomitus so that the patient should, if injuries permit, be positioned with his or her head on one side or in a semiprone position.

Sometimes, to control the bleeding, a nasogastric tube will be passed which in this case is the doctor's responsibility, and the stomach irrigated with cool normal saline in an attempt to create vasoconstriction and aid blood-clotting.

In all cases the degree of shock shown in the observations of blood pressure and pulse, and blood tests will indicate the treatment the patient will require for shock and the necessity or immediacy of surgery.

Control of Haemorrhage

Haemorrhage **must** be controlled. The treatment will depend upon the nature of the injury

For **external haemorrhage:**
  Apply direct pressure on wounds not containing glass or fragments.
  Apply indirect pressure with wounds containing glass or fragments.
  Elevate the affected area if a limb (see Chapter 4).

For **internal haemorrhage:**
  The extent must be assessed by observations (every 15 minutes) of blood pressure and pulse.

Blood Loss Replacement

Blood loss **must** be corrected by replacement. An intravenous infusion is commenced with plasma, dextran or whole blood when the blood group of the patient is determined.

Blood Groups

It is essential to determine a patient's blood group or type before giving blood to prevent the complication of incompatibility. Incompatibility means that the patient's blood reacts to the donor's blood and the donated red blood cells *(erythrocytes)*

clump together *(agglutination)*. This occurs in the capillaries, especially in the kidneys, leading to the eventual breakdown *(haemolysis)* of the erythrocytes.

Blood type or group is determined by the *antigen* present on the membrane of the erythrocyte. There are two main antigens known as A or B which divide blood groups into four types:

Those possessing A antigens only are Group A
Those possessing B antigens only are Group B
Those with both A and B antigens are Group AB
Those with no antigens are Group O

The percentage in the world population by group is:
A — 42 %; B — 9 %; AB — 3 %; and O — 46 %.

Related to the antigen are *antibodies* which are formed in response to the antigen and are found in the blood plasma. There are two antibodies or *agglutinins* related to the A and B antigens:

Alpha (α) or Anti a
Beta (β) or Anti b

Table 1 The antigen-antibody relationship.

Group	Antigen	Antibodies
A	A	Anti b
B	B	Anti a
AB	AB	None
O	O	Both anti a and anti b

Plasma never contains antibodies which would act against the antigens present in its own blood.

Another factor, the *rhesus factor*, which is an antigen formed on the erythrocyte, must be determined. Of the world population 85 % have this further antigen. If this factor is present, the blood type is rhesus positive (Rh +); if not present, it is rhesus negative (Rh −). This is important because a rhesus negative patient **cannot** be given rhesus positive blood as it would cause the reaction of agglutination.

The patient's blood type is determined by cross-matching. Cross-matching involves the donor's blood group being matched to the recipient's antibodies present in the plasma. The recipient's antibodies must not react to the donor's antigens. Group O blood does not have any antigens for the antibodies to react to, therefore, it can be given to all blood groups and is known as the *universal donor*. Because Group AB blood has both A and B antigens it cannot be given to the other groups as they all contain antibodies a and b. However, as group AB has no antibodies it can receive from all other blood groups, and is known as the *universal recipient*.

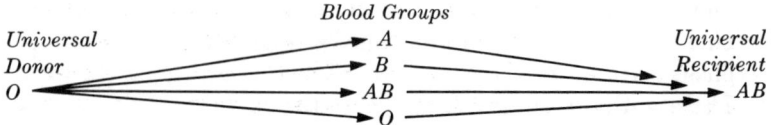

The arrows indicate the direction of donation. It must be remembered that each blood group can give and receive from its own group and this is the group of choice whenever possible. It must also be remembered that rhesus negative blood may be given to a rhesus positive patient.

```
Universal                                           Universal
Donor         ─────────────────────────▶            Recipient
O Rhesus negative                                   AB Rhesus positive
```

If the patient requires a rapid transfusion of blood a blood pump may be used. This pump creates a pressure on the bag of blood and forces it into the patient. In some hospitals a doctor must be present when a blood pump is in use.

Patient Care

Blood **must** circulate sufficiently to the vital organs. To enable the blood to circulate to the heart and brain of the patient in shock the nurse generally places the patient in the recumbent position with the foot of the trolley elevated. This is true except for patients who have:
Respiratory problems
Perforation of the bowel
In the latter case, the perforation allows bowel contents into the peritoneal cavity which might touch the diaphragm or liver and cause respiratory and liver problems.
The patient must be kept warm but not hot. If heat is applied to the patient it results in peripheral dilatation and removal of blood from the vital organs.
In the case of cardiogenic shock the heart action must be improved. Cardiogenic shock is generally caused by left

ventricular failure or myocardial infarction (see Chapter 5).
In vasodilative shock the aim is to produce vasoconstriction, for which the drug adrenaline is used.
Immediate surgery may be required in cases of uncontrolled or severe haemorrhage.

Administration of Analgesia for Shock

Analgesia is administered with extreme caution in conditions of shock. The body's reaction to *hypovolaemic* and *cardiogenic* shock is increased stimulation of the sympathetic nervous system resulting in peripheral vasoconstriction which assists in maintaining the blood pressure. Strong analgesia not only depresses the functioning of the central nervous system but also alters the effect of the sympathetic nervous system resulting in a change in vasoconstriction. In cases of cardiogenic shock, such as a myocardial infarction, patients are given strong analgesia (morphine). The reason why this is given is to allay the anxiety caused by the severe pain and to attempt to slow and steady the rate of the heart and respirations to create a more forceful and purposeful function.

Hypovolaemic Shock

In hypovolaemic shock the priority of treatment is to:
1 Maintain blood circulation to the vital organs
2 Control blood loss
3 Replace blood loss
Often analgesia is not given initially and the sympathetic vasoconstriction is allowed to aid blood-clotting.

Conclusions

The condition of shock **must** be recognized and treated accordingly.
It is an emergency.
The condition of shock can cause:
  Renal failure due to lack of blood circulating to the kidneys.
  Irreversible changes in tissue due to lack of oxygen, causing death.

UNCONSCIOUSNESS

For an unconscious patient the most important initial nursing care is maintaining an airway. Following this are observations of: breathing; circulation; and neurological function. General observation may indicate the cause of unconsciousness. When discussing the patient, the nurse and those in the immediate area should remember that in some levels of unconsciousness the patient can hear everything that is said.

Important observations to notify to the nurse or doctor in charge:
1 Deteriorating levels of consciousness
2 Increasing blood pressure
3 Decreasing pulse rate
4 Changes in pupil reaction
5 Leakage of cerebrospinal fluid from the nose or ears
6 Gross abnormality of temperature control

Please note that an unconscious patient may also have other changes in the blood pressure and pulse recordings. If the patient is suffering from severe haemorrhage following multiple injuries elsewhere in the body, he or she will produce the features of shock, i.e., hypotension and tachycardia.

Patient Care

The following points must be considered for care of the unconscious patient:
1 Maintenance of an airway.
2 Position of patient. An unconscious patient is generally nursed in a semiprone position but be aware of the patient's condition before he or she is moved to a semiprone position. A patient with spinal injuries, for instance, should be nursed in a recumbent position or a lateral position only, the spine must be kept straight during movement and at rest.
3 Movement of patient. If an unconscious patient remains in the accident and emergency department for any length of time his or her position must be changed every 2 hours to prevent the development of pressure sores. Observe any areas liable to pressure, noting any redness or breakdown of the skin.
4 Observations. These must be carried out at 15 minutes intervals.

5 Ensure that someone is with the unconscious patient at all times. Either nursing staff or a relative must be present to observe for any changes in the patient's condition.
6 Ensure that the sides of the trolley are always elevated when the patient is not being treated. Unconscious patients may move and this will prevent them from falling.
7 If the patient has been incontinent make sure that he or she is washed and dried thoroughly. If the urine is to be tested, especially in the case of a diabetic patient, prepare for catheterization.

Medical Intervention

The medical treatment is largely dependent on the cause (see Chapter 8). Signs of increasing intracranial pressure can be treated by drugs or surgery.

Drugs. If there is oedema of the brain cells due to the inflammatory response of the damaged cells drugs may be used:
 Dexamethasone — an anti-inflammatory steroid drug
 Frusemide (Lasix) or Mannitol — a diuretic

Surgery. Surgery may be used to relieve the pressure. Burr holes (holes through the skull) will relieve the haemorrhage which has occurred in the epidural or subdural region. However, the cause of raised intracranial pressure may be an abnormal growth within the brain. Neurosurgery may be able to remove, or partially remove, the growth to decrease the amount of pressure.

Care of the Patient Regaining Consciousness

The nurse **must** be alert to the fact that unconscious patients may regain consciousness at any time, and can often become confused, restless or even aggressive. At these times, the patient needs the nurse's professional sense of calmness, understanding and reassurance.
1 Explain simply, clearly and frequently to the patient where and why he or she is in the department, as the patient may be completely unaware of being brought there.
2 Stay with the patient to prevent any self-inflicted injury. If the patient is extremely restless ensure that you have enough

assistance to prevent such injury.
3   Avoid injury to yourself. This may not happen intentionally but the patient may not be in full control of his or her actions (see Chapter 11).
4   Ask the patient the reason for the restlessness. It may only be because of the discomfort being experienced, e.g., from a distended bladder and this may be relieved by allowing the patient to pass urine.
5   Be aware that the patient may have a headache or visual disturbances or may feel dizziness and nausea and may even vomit.

PAIN

Pain is a vital indication of the patient's condition and must be assessed accurately. The treatment of pain varies depending on other signs or symptoms of the pain.

Patient Care

When nursing a patient in pain remember that:
1   The relief of anxiety may alleviate pain to some extent. Quiet, reassuring words from you, explaining the treatment may reduce the general tension of the patient.
2   The positioning of the patient may give comfort and support, e.g., a suspected fracture should always be supported.
3   Keeping the patient warm will help to counteract the action of the sympathetic nervous system which in times of stress causes peripheral vasoconstriction. This vasoconstriction causes cold extremities and tenseness of muscles which aggravates pain stimuli.

Pain Relief

The relief of pain by drugs is the decision of the doctor and they **must** be used with caution. Pain and its effect on the sympathetic nervous system may be acting as a defence system for the patient, as it results in an increased blood pressure caused by general vasoconstriction. Relief of pain by strong analgesia may result in a sudden fall in the patient's blood pressure. Sympathetic stimulation also increases the respiratory rate, so relief of pain may cause severe respiratory depression as well.

Table 2 Drugs which can affect the peripheral or the central nervous system.

Peripheral nervous system	Central nervous system
Paracetamol (Panadol)	Papaveretum (Omnopon)
Aspirin	Pethidine hydrochloride
Dihydrocodeine	Morphine*
Codeine phosphate	

*Morphine is particularly useful in allaying the anxiety of a patient.

Removal of Causative Factors

To obtain relief from pain it may be necessary to remove the causative factor.
1 Reduction of fractures.
2 Manipulation of dislocations.
3 Removal of obstructions — surgery.
4 Removal of substance causing pain related with distension — nasogastric tube.
5 Reduction of inflammation, relieved by rest of affected area.
6 Administration of oxygen to the area of ischaemia, or cooling the area to decrease the amount of oxygen required.

Other Methods and Problems

Other methods of relieving pain involve the use of nerve blocks. There are accompanying problems with pain and these may be treated with drugs.
Nausea and vomiting — Anti-emetics, i.e., prochlorperazine (Stemetil) 12.5 mg, intramuscularly.
Muscle spam — Muscle relaxant, i.e., diazepam (Valium) 5-10 mg, intramuscularly.
Gastric irritation — Antacids, i.e., Gelusil 5-20 ml; Maalox 10-20 ml.

REVISION OBJECTIVES

At the end of this section the nurse learner will be able to discuss treatment in order of priority. This will include:
1 Maintaining a clear airway.
2 Assessing the patient's breathing.
3 Understanding the resuscitation procedure and the

principles of cardiac resuscitation.
4 Assisting with the taking of blood for blood gas estimations.
5 Making accurate observations of the respiratory function.
6 Administering oxygen.
7 Making accurate observations of the circulatory function.
8 Recognizing and controlling haemorrhage.
9 Understanding the relevance of blood groups to the administration of blood transfusions.
10 Caring for the unconscious patient.
11 Managing the patient who regains consciousness.
12 Describing the treatment of pain.

4
Minor Injuries

The majority of the work in an accident and emergency department is dealing with a multitude of minor injuries. The work is extremely interesting as it is very unlikely that there will be two patients in the department suffering from the same minor injury. This means that the nurses learn basic principles of care and then, using their own initiative, adapt each to the individual patient. It is while caring for these patients that nurse learners might find themselves following the doctor's orders to dress and bandage a lacerated wrist, but having to consider whether to apply a Crinx bandage or a crepe bandage; whether a sling will be necessary and what information will be needed by the patient in order to care for the injury. Nurses will also ensure that patients are informed as to whether there is a need to return for further treatment and, if so, when. When dealing with minor injuries nurses are not only caring for the patients in the department but instructing them on future care to ensure a safe recovery and to prevent complications.

INCISIONS AND LACERATIONS

An incision or cut is a clean straight opening of the skin. A laceration is an irregular, jagged cut. The former is the type of cut made during an operation or by a clean knife and the skin edges will come neatly together while the latter can be caused by a dirty object and the skin edges will not be neatly aligned.

Treatment

Treatment always involves an aseptic technique to ensure that the wound is kept as clean and free from bacteria as possible. The treatment will depend on:
  Depth of incision
  Length of incision
  Site of incision

Whether blood vessels are involved
Time at which incision occurred and length of time elapsed before the patient came to the accident and emergency department.

Depth of Incision. If the wound is deep and has gone into layers of subcutaneous fat and muscle causing the wound to gap then a dissolvable suture may be placed subcutaneously. Likewise if the skin edges do not come together easily to allow healing then skin sutures will be used to align the skin edges. There is a wide variety of skin sutures available. The choice of suture tends to vary with the site of the incision. Consequently the size of the needle and type of suture material vary. Where delicate areas of skin are sutured, such as on the face, a small needle and suture are used, e.g., No. 3 Silk. Where more tension is required on the wound edges, such as an incision which is going to be subject to movement, as on the fingers or knee, then a larger needle is used with a stronger suture, e.g., No. 4 Silk. However, the final choice of suture used is decided by the doctor performing the technique.

Suturing Equipment

The following equipment will need to be prepared for suturing:
    Clean surface
    Sterile pack containing:
        Gallipot for cleansing solution
        Sterile towel
        Swabs
        Gauze
        Toothed dissection forceps
        Nontoothed dissecting forceps
        Straight and curved mosquito forceps
        Needle holder
        Stitch scissors
    Local anaesthetic
    Syringes 2 ml and 5 ml for the anaesthetic
    Intramuscular and subcutaneous needles
    Suture material
    Adhesive tape or bandage for dressing
    Additional gauze for dressing

Suturing is not a nursing procedure but the nurse aids in the preparation of the equipment and care of the patient throughout the procedure, ensuring that the doctor's instructions for the aftercare are fully understood by the patient, relative or friend.

Length of Incision. The length of the incision will have a bearing on how easily the skin edges will come together, so that a short superficial wound does not always require suturing. However, this will vary according to the site of the wound.

Site of Incision. The site of the incision can determine its depth and whether it requires suturing. A wound on the hand may not be as deep as a wound on the abdomen but will be subject to a lot more movement and therefore a hindrance to wound healing, so sutures may be used for small wounds in areas of tension.

If the wound edges are in good apposition the application of butterfly sutures (plasters or steristrip dressing) across the wound edges to hold them together may be all that is required (Figure 7). These butterfly sutures should remain across the wound for the same length of time as a suture remains in position which is usually about 7 days. For a face wound which needs to heal without forming too much scar tissue, sutures are removed after 3 or 4 days.

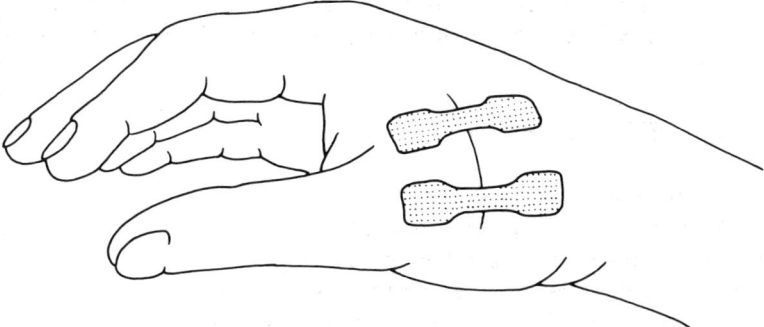

Figure 7 Steristrip dressing used to hold wound edges in apposition.

Wound Healing

Any opening into the skin surface creates a wound. The wound needs to heal quickly to prevent the complication of infection. Factors which influence good wound healing:
  Apposition of skin edges

Absence of dirt or infection
A good blood supply to skin edges

Other factors necessary are protein, vitamins A, and C. These aid in body building and cell repair and are obtained from a normal diet.

Stages of Wound Healing

The stages of wound healing involve the initial reaction to the injury and the repair following injury.

Reaction to injury
1 An inflammatory reaction which produces an increased blood supply to the area causing redness, swelling and heat.
2 The clotting mechanism which controls bleeding from damaged blood capillaries. The blood clot is formed within 4-5 minutes (see p.66).
3 An anti-inflammatory reaction. Bacteria and dead cells must be cleared away from the area. White blood cells *(leucocytes)* are required for this (see p.68).

Repair following injury
1 Collagen is formed by the growth of fibroblast cells within the blood clot. This initially forms granulation tissue and then scar tissue.
2 If the skin edges are in apposition then new epithelial tissue is formed by the epidermis growing across between the skin edges.

The initial healing process occurs within 3 days but good skin apposition and absence of bacteria can accentuate the healing process, this is known as *first intention healing*. *Second intention healing* takes longer and is a result of a loss of tissue and invasion of bacteria.

External Haemorrhage. If blood vessels are involved in the wound then bleeding must be controlled. This bleeding is called external haemorrhage as it can be seen by the observer. In the first aid situation direct or indirect pressure can be applied. This can also be applied in the casualty situation until the bleeding can be controlled. However the control of bleeding may require the intervention of the doctor.

Rules regarding the application of direct or indirect pressure:

Direct pressure can be applied in all instances except when there is suspected foreign material in the wound, especially glass, because by applying direct pressure the foreign material may recede further into the wound causing more damage. Direct pressure should always be applied with a clean material in the first aid station or with a sterile material in the accident and emergency department.

Indirect pressure may be applied in several ways (Figure 8).

By pressure on the appropriate arterial pressure point, e.g., facial, temporal, brachial, radial, or femoral.

By indirect pressure immediately around the wound using a dressing formed in the shape of a doughnut placed firmly around the wound and held in place by a bandage.

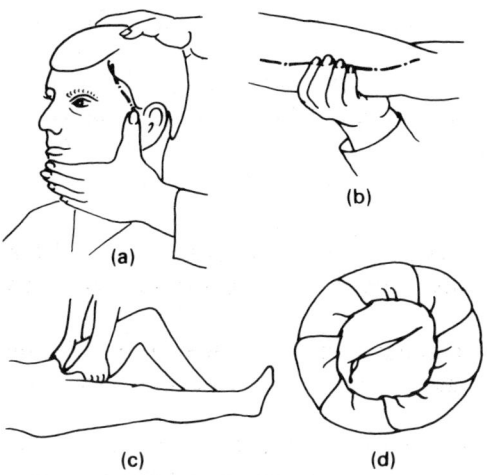

Figure 8 Means of controlling local bleeding: applying pressure to the temporal artery (a); applying pressure on the brachial artery of the arm (b); applying pressure to the femoral artery using both thumbs (c); applying indirect pressure: by means of a dressing immediately around a wound suspected of containing glass or a foreign object (d).

For wounds on the limbs, a tourniquet can be placed above the level of the injury (proximal to the injury). In the accident and emergency department an inflated sphygmomanometer cuff may be used, at a pressure above the radial pulse. This procedure should be used **only** when all other methods have been unsatisfactory. If a tourniquet is applied it must be released within 15 minutes to prevent tissue damage. A nurse applying a tourniquet **must** inform someone in authority, e.g., a doctor or a nurse that it has been applied.

In all cases of external haemorrhage elevating the affected area diminishes the blood supply to the wound and therefore limits blood loss.

Minor Injuries

Blood Clotting

Blood clotting is a natural control of bleeding. For bleeding to be controlled a series of chemical reactions must occur in a definite order. The substances involved are shown in Table 3.

Immediately after injury the blood supply to the area is reduced and local vasoconstriction occurs. This is produced by nerve reaction via the sympathetic nervous system.

The cut edge of the blood vessel produces a rough edge which causes the *platelets* circulating in the blood to adhere to the edge. These platelets produce *thromboplastin*, which starts the clotting mechanism, and begins to constrict the blood vessel.

Thromboplastin *(thrombokinase)* can only work in the presence of calcium, which is normally in the blood supply. The thromboplastin activates *prothrombin*, one of the plasma proteins normally circulating in the blood, to form thrombin.

Thrombin is now an active enzyme which can act on *fibrinogen* one of the circulating plasma proteins. Together they form *fibrin*. Fibrin is a fine network of threads which forms the blood clot by trapping blood cells.

Vitamin K is also needed for blood clotting. Although it can be obtained from the diet, it may be given intramuscularly to the patient. Vitamin K stimulates the cells of the liver to increase their production of prothrombin.

The normal bleeding time is 3-4 minutes. This depends on: constriction of the blood vessel and the clotting mechanism. Clotting time is 4-8 minutes.

Table 3   Substances involved in blood clotting.

Substances normally found in blood	Substances produced
Platelets	
Thromboplastin	
Calcium	Thrombin
Inactive prothrombin	
Fibrinogen	+ Thrombin = Fibrin

Time Since Injury. Wounds that have occurred within the last 12 hours are suitable for suturing if necessary.

Wounds that are more than 12 hours old have been exposed to the air and bacteria for a sufficient time to allow infection to enter. These are not sutured as this would hold the skin edges together and leave an area under the skin where infection could accumulate. Instead these wounds are allowed to granulate from the bottom. They are kept as clean as possible by aseptic dressings with butterfly skin sutures holding the skin edges in close apposition.

Cleaning a Wound

It is necessary to remove any grease, dirt or suspected foreign bodies from the wound and the immediate surrounding area and to locate the area of the wound if there is haemorrhage.

Oil, Grease or Dirt. With hand injuries, patients with oil, grease or dirt on their hands are advised to wash around the injured area with soap and water or special hand-cleansing cream, **except** when there is external bleeding which needs to be controlled.

In other cases or after the patient has washed the area, the wound is cleaned using an aseptic technique with aseptic solutions such as Savlon or eusol.

Foreign Bodies. If there is a suspected foreign body in the wound then the wound can be immersed in hydrogen peroxide. Remember that hydrogen peroxide bubbles up during its reaction so the patient **must** be protected against spillage from the container.

Haemorrhage. In wounds that have caused haemorrhage it is important to find the site of the wound and the bleeding. In the case of scalp wounds this can be difficult and there is sometimes considerable haemorrhage. When possible the wound should be located and clean the area moving away from the wound edges thereby limiting the risk of infection.

It must be remembered that the sight of blood to the patient, friends or relatives can be very distressing. Once the patient is cleaned up it can often be seen that the bleeding has come from a small wound though the initial impression was of more severe trauma. The patient must be reassured and accompanying friends or relatives allowed to visit the patient after the bleeding has been controlled and the patient cleaned up.

PUNCTURE WOUND

A puncture wound has a very small opening with minimal damage to the epidermis of the skin, sometimes hardly visible to the naked eye, but is deep. It can be caused by a sharp pointed instrument such as a nail or a knife.

Treatment

The care of a puncture wound varies depending on its position but the main concerns are internal damage and the risk of the introduction of infection (see Chapter 9).

Puncture wounds which involve damage only to the skin structures can be dealt with as minor injuries. It is important to ensure by X-ray that all of the object has been removed from the skin, such as a nail, a drawing pin or a splinter of glass. Hydrogen peroxide can be used to remove the object or, if necessary, the doctor may need to incise the wound surgically to take out the object. Whichever way the wound is treated it must be cleaned aseptically and dressed. The patient **must** be advised to be aware of signs of infection and may be treated conservatively with a course of antibiotics or given tetanus toxoid (see p.80).

If the object is still within the wound it will produce an inflammatory reaction leading to infection.

Inflammatory Reaction

The inflammatory reaction is the first response of the body to injury or the presence of foreign material. The reaction in the case of injury to the skin is very closely related to the blood clotting mechanism, afore mentioned, and assists in wound healing.

The reaction in cases of infection is against bacteria. It is the leucocytes that are responsible for the reaction of the body to bacteria (foreign material). Leucocytes can be divided into two main groups: *granulocytes* and *agranulocytes*.

The inflammatory response concerns the granulocytes. There are three types of granulocytes, but the ones concerned with the initial inflammatory wound response are the neutrophils.

Neutrophils are phagocytic cells and engulf bacteria. They are the first leucocytes at the site of injury or inflammation and they adhere to the walls of the blood vessels, which have become sticky. They then force themselves out of the capillary into the surrounding damaged tissue where they commence their activity. As the neutrophils die they form pus which also contains dead bacteria.

Other granulocytes involved in the inflammatory response are the *monocytes* which are large phagocytic cells belonging to the group of mononuclear cells. These cells arrive at the site of inflammation at the later stage and develop into *macrophages*. They clear the bacteria from the area and they may continue this function for several months.

Summary of an Infection

Initially an infection begins with the invasion of bacteria, followed by the inflammatory response.

Inflammatory response:
1   Local vasodilation often assisted by the release of histamine. This may be produced by the leucocytes known as *basophils*.
2   Cells and fluid filter from the blood vessels into the surrounding tissue and produce swelling. The increased blood supply produces redness and heat.
3   Neutrophils begin their action.
4   Macrophages complete the action.
5   Pus is produced. If this forms under the epithelium of the skin then an abscess will be formed and will require evacuation.
6   Pain may be produced by the effect of stimulation of foreign substances on local nerve endings.

ABRASION

Abrasion is the loss of a thin layer of skin and, depending on the depth of the grazing, can leave small capillaries exposed, causing superficial bleeding. Abrasions usually heal quickly as long as the area is kept free of infection.

Treatment

The area is cleaned with a cleaning solution and either left exposed, or dressed. Facial abrasions are left **exposed** and can be cleaned with sterile water at 2-hourly intervals to keep the skin supple and free from infection. When **dressing** abrasions it must be remembered that the superficial bleeding and the healing process will adhere to surrounding materials so apply non adherent dressings to any wound which will produce oozing. This prevents trauma to the patient's skin when the dressing is removed and the wound exudate has hardened. There are several non adherent dressings, e.g., Melolin, and nurses must be sure to know the preference of their department.

If the abrasion has been caused by a dirty object then a dressing containing an antibiotic may be applied directly to the wound. The following dressings have an oily base such as petroleum jelly to prevent adherence to the wound:

    Jelonet

    Bactigras — this contains an antiseptic, chlorhexidine.

    Sofratulle — this contains an antibiotic, framycetin sulphate 1%.

MINOR BURNS

A burn is an injury to the tissues caused by physical, chemical or electrical agents.

Minor or superficial burns produce skin redness, tissue damage, blistering, a risk of infection and possible deformity. Superficial burns are also very painful, although not deep.

FIRST AID MEASURES

The actions in first aid treatment for a burn are:

1 Immerse area or limb in cold water or under running water. This lessens the pain and decreases peripheral circulation thus limiting the amount of plasma loss from the burnt area. If the burn is caused by a chemical, wash or irrigate the chemical away from the skin.

2 Remove any local jewellery such as watches, rings or chains as the area might become swollen and then the objects may have to be cut off.

3 Remove any clothing from the area if it is not adhering to the burnt area, and loosely wrap the area in a clean object e.g., a pillow case.

4 Transport person to an accident and emergency department.

Treatment

On arrival in the department the patient must be treated for pain as well as for the burnt area. **Remember** in the case of a child who has received minor burns both the child and the accompanying parent or guardian will be distressed.
Remove clothing or items of jewellery, if they have not already been removed.
Prepare a trolley for an aseptic technique as the burnt area will be cleaned (Savlon) and dressed, after the doctor examines it.

Equipment for Aseptic Technique

Equipment needed for a basic aseptic technique includes:
Clean surface
Sterile pack containing:
  Gallipot
  Swabs
  Gauze
  Sterile towel
Forceps
Cleaning solution, e.g., Savlon
Adhesive tape for dressing or appropriate bandage to hold dressing in place.
Scissors for cutting tape
Additional dressing if required

If a blister has formed the doctor may order that it is evacuated or removed. This can be done by either the nurse or the doctor using a sterile needle or sterile scissors to pierce or cut the blister away. Sterile swabs are used to apply pressure on the blister and to remove the exudate.

If the area is cleaned with Savlon, **remember** to work towards the dirty area from the clean area and from the burnt area to the surrounding intact skin. This procedure usually soothes the patient's skin to some extent. However, it is important to ensure that the doctor prescribes analgesia if necessary before the procedure and that the patient has analgesia available at home.

Due to prescription cost, it is advisable to suggest to the patient the purchase of an appropriate analgesia, e.g., Panadol or soluble aspirin, from a local chemist.

Once the area has been cleaned it can be dressed with non adherent dressings or a soothing antibiotic cream such as

Flamazine. Burns can also be dressed with a sterile covering sheet of Op-Site. This sheet allows the burn to heal without the risk of the introduction of infection and allows easy observation of the site while the dressing is in place.

To prevent further damage to the skin following a burn the dressing is usually held in place by a bulky bandage with padding. If it is the hand area that is to be bandaged it is particularly important, as in all bandages over joints, to hold the joint in a position of extension. This prevents the complication of contractions. A hand, for instance, may be dressed with padding in the palm so that the fingers are extended, alternatively, the hand may be dressed with Flamazine and placed in a plastic bag. This keeps the hand clean but allows for finger movement to prevent contractions.

Burns to the face are not usually dressed but left exposed having been treated with Povidone iodine. The patient, relative or friend must be instructed to apply this every 2 – 3 hours if the patient is discharged.

ABSCESS

An abscess is an advanced stage of inflammation where pus has collected as a result of infection by bacteria. This is not always caused by trauma but does result from bacteria entering the skin. The cause of an abscess may have been an insect bite or from an infected hair follicle. However, whatever the cause the inflammatory response will have commenced and, in the case of an abscess, the pus is contained within healthy tissue where healing cannot occur until the pus is removed and the skin edges allowed to granulate.

The patient will complain of pain and discomfort from the abscess. It will be warm and tender to touch. Other accompanying symptoms can be a raised temperature due to the infection, although in an abscess the infection is generally localized to the area. Depending on the site of the abscess, the patient may be reluctant to move the area affected, e.g., the arm, if the abscess is in the axilla.

Treatment

Treatment in accident and emergency department involves the

removal of the pus and bacteria to allow healing.
1   A closed abscess can be treated with a glycerine and ichthammol dressing.
2   An open abscess can be cleaned aseptically and then dressed with a solution of magnesium sulphate. Magnesium sulphate has an osmotic effect and will draw water towards it and therefore draws the pus to the surface of the skin.
3   The abscess can be surgically incised aseptically and the pus removed. If this is done the nurse must prepare the patient and the necessary equipment.

Equipment for Incision and Drainage

The equipment needed for incision and drainage of an abcess:
   Clean surface
   Sterile pack containing:
      2 gallipots: one for cleansing solution and one for packing solution, e.g., eusol and paraffin.
      Sterile towel
      Swabs
      Gauze
      Probe
      Nontoothed dissecting forceps
      Sinus forceps
      Stitch scissors
      Curved mosquito forceps
      Volkman spoon
      A swab for culture and sensitivity

This is not a comfortable procedure for a patient so that analgesia must be considered. The usual choice in the case of an abscess for incision and drainage is a spray-on local anaesthetic such as lignocaine hydrochloride. However, if the abscess is particularly large and painful, the patient may receive Entonox, (see Chapter 9) or may require a general anaesthetic.

Preoperative Care

If the patient requires a general anaesthetic it must be remembered that preoperative care must be carried out as follows:
1   Ensure that the patient signs a consent form. (If he or she is under 16 years of age then the consent form should be signed by a parent or legal guardian).

2 Determine when the patient last had anything by mouth. It is legally required, except in an emergency, that a patient has had nothing by mouth for 4 - 6 hours prior to surgery.
3 Contact the anaesthetist to see the patient.
4 Prepare the patient by:
Placing the patient in an operation gown.
Allowing the patient to pass urine.
Removing any prosthesis such as dentures or contact lenses.
Placing an identification bracelet on the patient's wrist.

Notify the next of kin, relative or friend so that someone is available to escort the patient home when his or her condition is satisfactory.

It is important to reassure the patient and explain the procedure, remembering that the patient may only have come into the department because of a painful lump, e.g., in the axilla, and would not be expecting to undergo an operation.

Once the patient and equipment have been prepared then the doctor will complete the procedure.

Administration of Anaesthesia

The anaesthetist will administer the anaesthetic. Thiopentone sodium is given intravenously and takes effect within 10-30 seconds producing loss of consciousness for 2-3 minutes. The patient is given oxygen at this time and then an intraveous injection of suxamethonium chloride (Scoline). Scoline is a short-acting muscle relaxant which would allow the anaesthetist to pass an endotracheal tube if required. A tube is not usually required as the anaesthesia is usually administered by mask in the accident and emergency department. By mask, the patient is kept anaesthetised by a mixture of gas, oxygen and halothane.

Stages of Anaesthesia. There are 4 stages of anaesthesia:
1 Analgesia — The patient is awake, aware and co-operative (see section on Entonox).
2 Excitement — The patient is asleep and unaware of his or her actions. There is a release of inhibitions and the patient may become extremely restless.
3 Surgical anaesthesia — Surgery may be performed during this stage, which is composed of 4 levels.

4 Failure of vital functions — The respiratory system is depressed and the patient requires ventilation. The circulatory system is depressed causing hypotension and eventually cardiac arrest.

Patient Care

During the administration of the anaesthesia the nurse can ensure the patient's safety, especially as the patient goes into the second stage of anaesthesia when there is rapid muscular contraction. Standing by the side of the operating table the nurse can steady the patient's arms, legs and body.

If an anaesthetic is administered in the accident and emergency department the patient will just be put into the third stage as the anaesthetic is generally only required for a short period and will be administered via a mask. The patient is observed afterwards until consciousness returns and the swallowing reflex is present.

During the procedure the nurse can assist the doctor and also be responsible for taking a wound swab as soon as the doctor has incised the abscess. On completion of the procedure the nurse is usually responsible for dressing the area and for the recovery of the patient.

Postoperative Care

As with all postoperative patients the same important factors must be considered:

Maintenance of an Airway. On completion of the procedure, the patient is usually nursed in a semiprone position to maintain the airway. An airway may be *in situ*, but the patient is encouraged to push this out as soon as consciousness is regained.

Assessment of Breathing. The anaesthetist will assess the patient's breathing and ensure that the patient is breathing spontaneously on completion of the procedure. It is then the nurse's responsibility to observe and assess the patient's breathing until the patient is well enough to leave the department.

Observation of the Cardiovascular System. Record the pulse every 15 minutes as it is an accurate assessment of the cardiovascular system. It is not usually necessary to take a patient's blood pressure.

Dressing Care. Care should be taken of the incision dressing as follows:

There might be some oozing as the purpose of the procedure was to evacuate an abscess, but the oozing should be serosanguineous fluid and pus, **not** fresh blood. If there is a lot of oozing following the procedure then the wound may need to be re-dressed before the patient is discharged.

The patient may have had a gauze wick or packing put into the incised abscess during the procedure. The gauze is usually soaked in eusol and paraffin. The eusol is used to clean the wound of bacteria; the paraffin to keep the gauze moist and prevent it drying out and adhering to the walls of the abscess.

The gauze used for packing an abscess must be radiopaque (this is shown by the blue line in the gauze) and it ensures that if packing is lost in a patient it can be located on X-ray. To prevent gauze being left in a patient's abscess cavity only one piece of gauze should be packed into the cavity and a small piece at the end left on the outside of the abscess.

The pack serves two purposes, one to allow the cavity to granulate from the bottom towards the skin surface (if the skin surfaces were allowed to come together before the bottom of the cavity had healed then an abscess would form again). Secondly, the packing also allows drainage of the abscess because it has created an opening to the skin surface.

Instructions for the Patient

If the patient has a pack in place then it is essential for instructions to be given as to when and where to go to have the pack removed and a new one inserted if necessary. The usual care is for the patient to return daily for re-dressing either to the accident and emergency department or to the health centre, in which case the general practitioner must be notified and a letter sent with the patient explaining what has been administered in the casualty department.

If the abscess has been treated with magnesium sulphate dressings then the patient may return every two or three days for re-application or for incision and dressing.

When skin sutures or butterfly sutures have been used, the patient will be asked to return to the accident and emergency department or the doctor for removal of these.

Facial sutures are removed afer 4 days and other sutures after 7 days.

If the patient is attending his or her own general practitioner make sure that there is an accompanying doctor's letter.

With some butterfly sutures, the patient may be instructed to remove them only returning to the general practitioner or the department if any problems arise. It is necessary to make sure that before a patient leaves the department that the care of the injury is properly understood. These instructions can be given verbally to the patient, relative or friend or can be given in writing.

If the patient is unable to make the journey to the hospital or health centre then the nurse must either arrange transport, e.g., an ambulance, to bring the patient to the hospital at the appropriate time or arrange for the district nurse to visit and treat the patient at home.

DRESSINGS

The injuries mentioned are the types of minor injuries encountered in hospital requiring an aseptic technique and some form of dressing. These injuries require a secure dressing that will not hinder movement too much remembering that most of these patients will be returning to work.

Bandages used are generally:
1   Crinx bandages — do not cause compression on the area.
2   Strapping — it must be first ascertained that the patient is not allergic to this type.
3   Elastic net surgical tubular stockinette (Netalast), especially for dressings in the axilla, on the back or on the buttocks (Figure 9).

Each dressing will differ in some way so the nurse's care must be adapted to the individual patient.

Tubinette

Dressings on the fingers and the toes can be held in place by using a tubinette dressing.

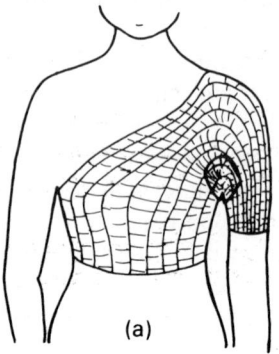
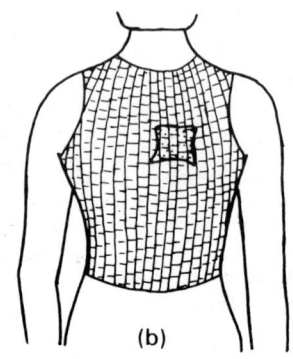
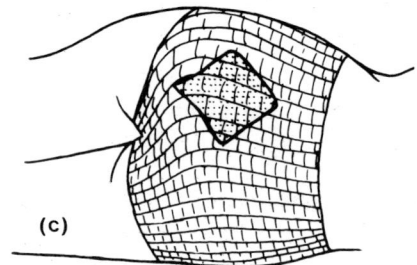

Figure 9 Netalast used to hold dressings in place: in the axilla (a); on the chest or back (b); on the buttocks (c).

Requirements:
 Small tubinette on finger applicator
 Scissors

Application:
1 Follow aseptic technique. After the aseptic technique, wherever there may be exudate (oozing) from the wound, apply non adherent dressings before the tape or bandage.
2 Place gauze dressing loosely around finger.
3 Apply a small amount of tape if necessary but do not make a tight dressing.
4 Use finger applicator with tubinette of appropriate length.
5 Place applicator over dressing and slide end of tubinette onto finger and hold in position. (Figure 10a).
6 Move applicator off finger and twist around so that tubinette twists at top of finger or toe. (Figure 10b).

7 Push applicator over finger again and slide off end of tubinette onto finger. (Figure 10c).
8 Remove applicator again and twist round. Do this procedure three or four times then remove applicator.
9 Hold out tubinette and cut down centre (Figure 10d) and then tie around the wrist, ensuring that the patient can bend the finger, or secure loosely around base of finger or toes (Figure 10e).

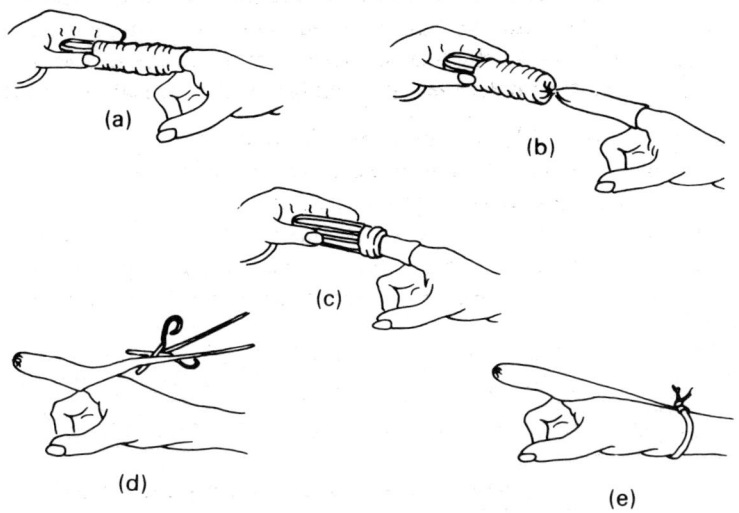

Figure 10 Application of a finger dressing: the applicator is placed over the dressing and the end of the tubinette is slid onto the injured figure (a), and the applicator is moved off the finger and the tubinette twisted (b). This procedure is repeated several times (c), and the remaining tubinette is cut down the centre (d), and tied around the wrist (e).

Instructions for the Patient

After a dressing has been applied, inform the patient that:
1 The dressing must be kept dry and intact. The patient may require to wear plastic gloves if the dressing is on the hand in order that work may be continued, i.e., if the patient is a butcher or a mechanic. However, warmth is generated inside a plastic or waterproof glove and this creates an ideal environment for bacteria. So if a patient needs to wear gloves in order to continue work then it must be emphasized that the gloves must be worn no longer than necessary and removed at frequent intervals.

Minor Injuries

2 If the dressing becomes soiled or wet then it should be re-applied, either by the patient if able (the nurse must decide this) or the patient must return to the department for the wound to be re-dressed.
3 The affected area must be gently exercised, especially if the injury has occurred near a joint, such as the fingers, elbows or knees.
4 If the affected area becomes hot and more painful, or, in the case of fingers and toes, it becomes hot and throbs painfully, the patient should return to his or her doctor or to the department.
5 The patient must be informed as to when and where to return for follow-up care (see p. 77).

CARE OF MINOR INJURIES

Prevention of Infection

For the prevention of infection to minor injuries it is necessary to note:

An aseptic technique prevents the introduction of any additional bacteria, and helps eliminate bacteria if present. Keeping the wound dry and covered with sterile material prevents the introduction of bacteria.

Local application of antibiotics such as those found in paraffin gauze helps destroy bacteria present.

Systemic administration of antibiotics. The initial dose of these antibiotics may be given intramuscularly to the patient in the accident and emergency department if there is a suspected risk of infection.

Administration of Antibiotics

When giving an antibiotic it is vital to assess whether the patient is allergic to antibiotics. If the patient is under 16 years of age then parental or guardian consent must be obtained.

It is advisable to observe the patient for a period of 15 minutes after the administration of an antibiotic because if the patient does become allergic to the drug the condition of *anaphylactic shock* will develop and **immediate** treatment will be required. This situation arises very rarely but, due to its severity, the nurse must be aware of a patient's reaction to antibiotics.

Administration of Tetanus Toxoid

For protection against infection caused by the bacteria *Clostridium tetani* tetanus toxoid is administered. This bacteria is found in the intestines of some animals, especially horses, and results in the condition of tetanus.

In favourable conditions the bacteria form spores which are often found in soil and so many minor injuries are contaminated with the *Clostridium tetani* bacteria. The spores do not themselves produce an infection but they produce a toxin. The toxin affects the spinal cord, having travelled along the nerve to the cord. It then inhibits controlling impulses to the muscles, so the muscles are over stimulated and react by convulsive twitching or continual contraction. The first symptom of the condition may occur in the jaw muscles hence tetanus has become known as lock jaw, but any group of muscles may be affected in this way. The main complications of the condition are exhaustion and inability to control breathing. The condition can develop anytime from a few days to a month from the time of the original injury.

It is important to ensure that each patient has some immunity to the disease because of its severity. Consequently, each patient who has received a minor injury is asked about vaccinations against tetanus during the last 3-5 years. The usual dosage is 0.5 mg tetanus toxoid.

Children are often protected from tetanus because tetanus toxoid is given with their immunisation at ages 3, 6 and 12 months, and 5 years.

If the patient has not been vaccinated against tetanus within the last 3-5 years then a course of injections must be commenced. The course consists of 3 injections, the first being given while the patient is in casualty, the second in 6 months time and the third within a year. The patient must understand that successful immunity to tetanus is not achieved until the three injections are given, but in the meantime only a temporary immunity is provided.

The patient is advised to return to his or her general practitioner for the second and third injections thereby limiting the work of the accident and emergency department. The patient should be issued with a card, stating when to return for follow-up injections and told the importance of showing the card on any further injury.

If the patient has had an injection of tetanus toxoid within the last 3-5 years but not in the last year then a booster injection will be given. This consists of one injection of 0.5 mg tetanus toxoid. It is important for a patient to remember when the last tetanus injection was given as this prevents a course being given unnecessarily. The tetanus toxoid injection can be administered subcutaneously or intramuscularly. With seriously contaminated wounds, a patient who has never had established immunity against tetanus may be given Humotet, an antitetanus immunoglobulin injection along with the tetanus toxoid.

Instructions for the Patient

Other care involves advising the patient to report to the doctor or the department if signs of infection become obvious. The patient should be alert to:

Increasing pain in the wound or a throbbing sensation — this occurs especially in the fingers.
Redness of the wound
Swelling of the wound
Increasing skin heat around the wound
Oozing from the wound. In the case of an abscess a patient should be warned that this can be expected but oozing through the dressing requires re-dressing.

It is not only nursing and medical management of a patient that prevents the complication of infection but the patient's awareness and care of the wound, so the patient must be instructed carefully.

Exercise

It is important to advise all patients to gently exercise the injured area regularly. Although the patient has only received a minor injury, if the affected digit or limb is not moved for a period of 7 to 10 days but is held stiff with the muscles contracted, the result can mean that the patient requires physiotherapy to relax the affected muscles. This can prolong a patient's rehabilitation.

Obstruction of Blood Supply

Blood supply obstruction may result from direct injury at the time of trauma and leave some tissue without a blood supply. This will lead to *necrosis* (tissue death) of the area. If this is suspected then the patient must return to the doctor or to the department for regular observation of the wound. The dead tissue, usually a small area in minor injuries, will eventually have to be removed for the healthy tissue to granulate from below.

Unfortunately the incorrect application of dressings and bandages may lead to the complication of an obstructed blood supply especially of the fingers. It must be remembered that when a dressing is applied it is held in place by a non compressive bandage. The bandage should not be tight enough to constrict the blood supply. The patient must always be asked if the dressing is comfortable.

DISCHARGING A PATIENT

When discharging a patient from the department, stop and think. Ensure that the patient is dressed to leave the department, understands care of the injury, and has a prescription if necessary.

Leaving the Department. Ensure that the patient is able to leave department. For instance, are clothes such as a pair of trousers which have had to be cut off or a heavily blood-stained blouse which was removed, suitable for wearing again? If shoes cannot be worn provide alternative footwear, e.g., plaster boots. Make sure that the patient is decently dressed. These considerations might appear to be obvious but in a busy department when one patient after another requires treatment it may not be realised or noticed that a patient has had to hop from the department because a shoe will not fit over an injured foot or another patient may be leaving on a very cold day dressed only in a shirt and trousers because of being brought in by a workmate who did not wait.

Ensure that the patient can be supported or taken by wheelchair out to a car to be taken home.

Care of Injury. If the patient cannot bear weight on an injured foot provide a walking stick or crutches and instruct the patient on the use of these (see p.94).

Minor Injuries 83

If the patient requires a sling to elevate an injured arm then this must be provided. Make sure the patient can cope with any personal property. The injury may have been sustained when out shopping and the patient may not be able to carry this home.

Ensure that the patient has any follow-up instructions and knows and understands how to care for the wound.

Check with the doctor whether the patient can return to work.

See whether a sick note is required for work and make sure that this is completed by the doctor and given to the patient.

Drugs by Prescription. If the patient requires drugs by prescription make sure the prescription is given and check whether the patient has enough money to pay for it.

Advise the patient where the prescription can be obtained.

At the times when hospital pharmacies and chemists are not open the department may need to issue enough tablets for the patient until such time as the prescription can be used.

Do not send a patient home in obvious pain without ensuring that the patient has some analgesia.

STRAINS, SPRAINS AND FRACTURES

Minor injuries with a visible wound have already been mentioned but there are other injuries which do not always have external wounds and may require supportive bandages. Such injuries include strains, sprains and fractures.

A **strain** is the stretching of a part of the body, e.g., a tendon or a muscle.

A **sprain** is a painful injury to a joint which causes swelling. Movement of the joint is often reduced because of the pain. The injury has involved tearing of the ligaments attached to the bone. This condition can often present as a fracture and only an X-ray will show the exact state of the injury.

A **fracture** is a broken bone. Not all fractures come under the heading of minor injuries (see Chapter 9) but some, e.g., fractures of the phalanges or a fractured clavicle, are counted as minor and the patient treated and discharged home.

Treatment

Supportive Bandages

Strains and sprains may be treated with supportive bandaging. In some cases the bandages provide compression so great care must be taken not to constrict the blood supply.

Nurses must be aware of the materials and techniques used in the particular department in which they are working as these vary in different departments.

Bandages which can be applied to various injuries: a thumb spica, a finger splint, a ring strapping, an arm or leg strapping, a collar and cuff sling, a Robert Jones bandage, and a sling (if the patient requires a sling following an injury to an arm or to the shoulder).

Thumb Spica. A thumb spica is applied to support the thumb is a neutral position following a sprain or other injury.

Requirements:
 Tubinette
 Elastoplast, 2.5 cm

Application:
1 Place the tubinette over the hand and thumb.
2 Using Elastoplast and starting below the distal interphal-

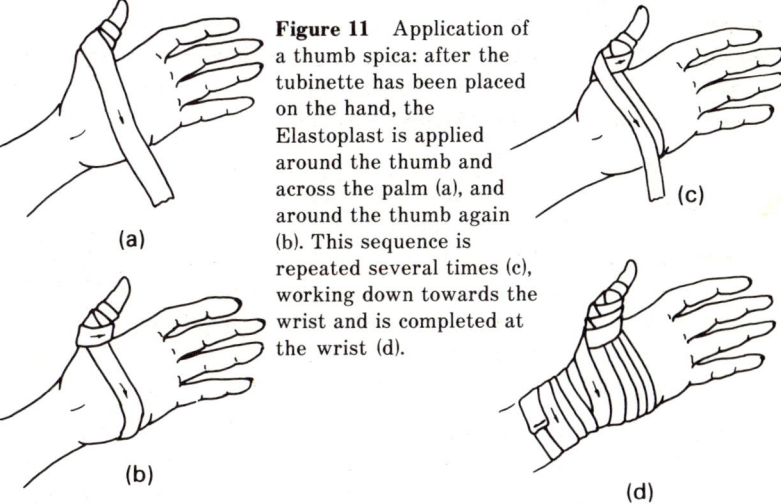

Figure 11 Application of a thumb spica: after the tubinette has been placed on the hand, the Elastoplast is applied around the thumb and across the palm (a), and around the thumb again (b). This sequence is repeated several times (c), working down towards the wrist and is completed at the wrist (d).

Minor Injuries

angeal joint, apply 2 turns around the thumb. On the left thumb apply the Elastoplast anticlockwise; on the right thumb clockwise (Figure 11a).
3 Bring the plaster straight across the palm, around the thumb itself and back again across the palm (Figure 11b).
4 Repeat the entire sequence for 3 or 4 complete turns (Figure 11c) overlapping each turn by at least half to work down the thumb and down the palm towards the wrist.
5 Ensure that while applying the dressing the thumb is in the neutral position and can bend inwards.
6 Take one further layer across the base of the palm and finish with 2 or 3 complete turns around the wrist (Figure 11d).

Instructions for the patient:
1 The dressing is to remain in position for 10 days or until the follow-up appointment.
2 Try to avoid getting the dressing wet.
3 Keep the hand elevated if any swelling presents.
4 Exercise the thumb by gentle movement in towards the hand.
5 Return to your doctor, if the hand becomes swollen or the dressing becomes tight. If the thumb becomes white, cold or blue, remove the bandages and return to your doctor

Finger Splint. A finger splint is applied to immobilize a fracture of the phalanges.

Requirements:
  Finger splint
  Zinc oxide tape or Elastoplast, 2.5 cm

Application:
1 Measure the finger splint from the wrist over the finger to the base of the finger—bend the splint and break at the appropriate length.
2 Fold back the ends of the splint. Bend into shape over the finger maintaining the finger in the neutral position.
3 Tape the splint in place (Figure 12).

Instructions for the patient:
1 Remember to exercise the other fingers.
2 If the hand or finger is swollen, keep the hand elevated whenever possible.
3 Return to your doctor or the fracture clinic as indicated.

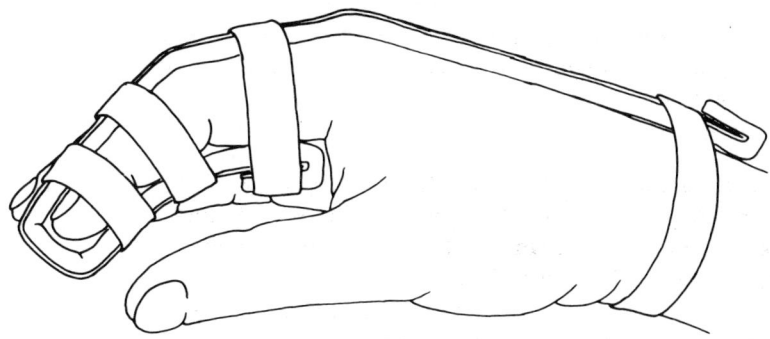

Figure 12 A zimmer splint in position. **Note** the ends of the splint are folded back to prevent any injury to the patient.

Ring Strapping. A ring strapping is applied to immobilize and give support to an injured digit.

Requirements:
   Piece of gauze or tubinette
   Zinc oxide tape, 1.75 cm or 2.5 cm

Application:
1 Place the gauze between the affected digit and the next digit (Figure 13a) or place the tubinette over these 2 digits (Figure 13b).
2 Place strapping around both digits between the joints (Figure 13c).

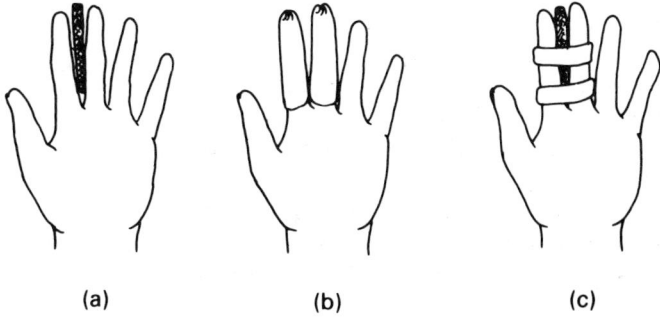

Figure 13 Application of a ring strapping: place gauze between the affected digits (a), or place tubinette over them (b). Strapping is then applied around the digits (c).

Instructions for the patient:
1 The uninjured digit is acting as a splint or support to the injured one but the fingers or toes should still be moved by bending when possible.
2 Return to the fracture clinic if an appointment is given.
3 Return to your doctor if there is excessive swelling or a throbbing pain.

Strapping. A strapping is applied to support the limb after a non-fracture injury.

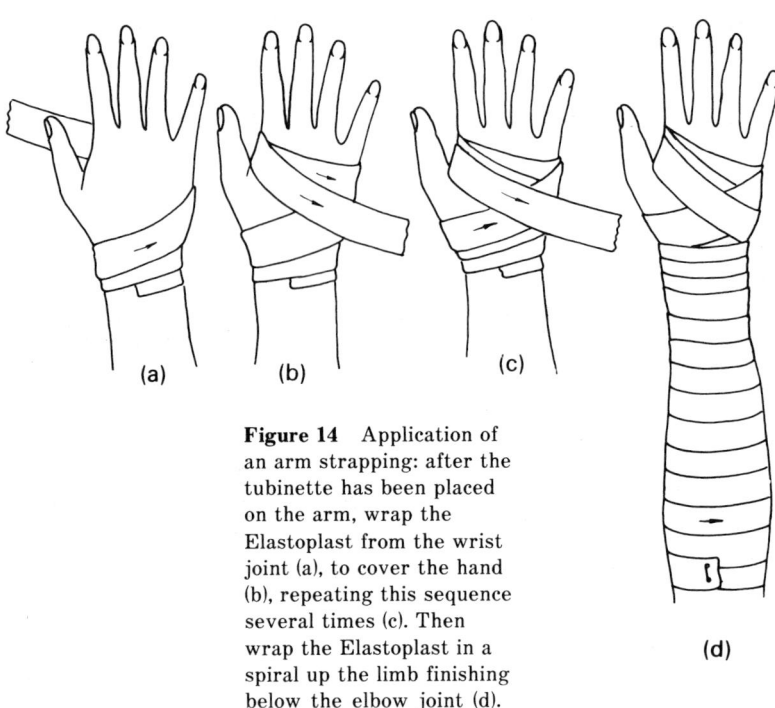

Figure 14 Application of an arm strapping: after the tubinette has been placed on the arm, wrap the Elastoplast from the wrist joint (a), to cover the hand (b), repeating this sequence several times (c). Then wrap the Elastoplast in a spiral up the limb finishing below the elbow joint (d).

Requirements:
  Stockinette
  Elastoplast

Application:
1 Cut the stockinette into an appropriate length, i.e., from the ankle to the knee; from the wrist to the elbow.

2   Wrap the Elastoplast from the joint — wrist (Figure 14a) or foot (Figure 15a) — from the inside to the outside of the limb covering the hand or foot. Stretch the Elastoplast before applying.
3   This sequence is repeated several times (Figure 14b and Figure 15b).
4   Wrap in a spiral up the limb (Figure 14c and 15c) covering half of the bandage at each turn.
5   Fix the top of the bandage over the skin to hold the bandage in place, making sure that the strapping covers the limb from joint to joint, on the arm to below the elbow joint, on the leg to 2.5 cm below the popliteal tendon (Figure 14d and 15d).

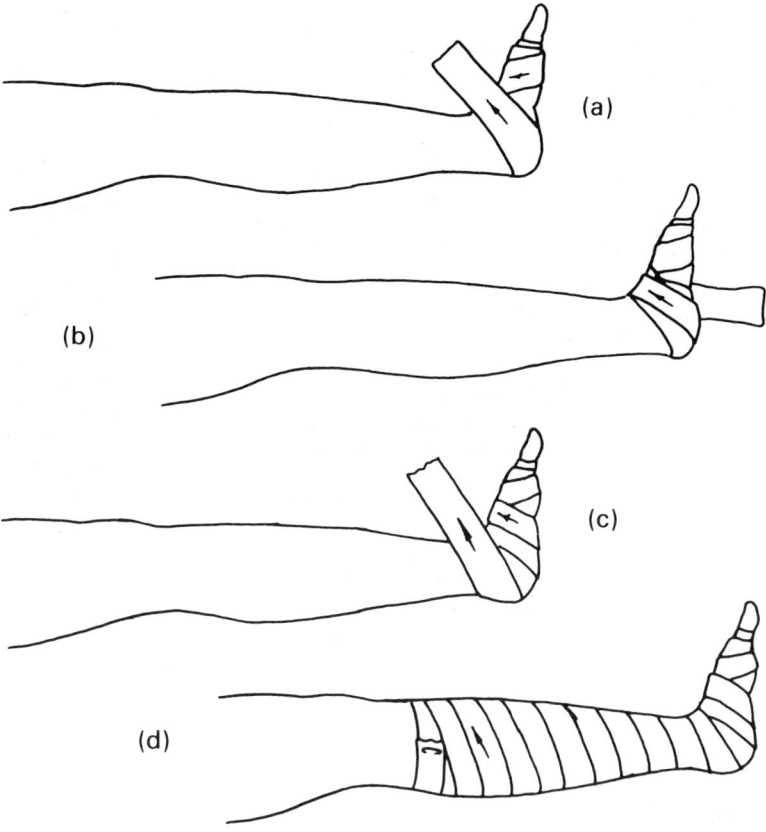

Figure 15   Application of a leg strapping: after the tubinette has been applied, wrap the Elastoplast from the ankle joint (a), to cover the foot (b), and repeat this procedure several times (c). Then wrap the Elastoplast in a spiral up the limb finishing below the knee joint (d).

Instructions for the patient:
1 Strapping is applied to support a limb and is to remain in place for 10 days or until the follow-up appointment.
2 If the strapping becomes too tight or the fingers turn blue, white or cold, remove the bandage and return to your doctor.
3 Keep the limb elevated to prevent any swelling.

Collar and Cuff Sling. A collar and cuff sling is provided to rest the limb or to support the limb following trauma to the shoulder or in the case of a fractured humerus. It is an alternative to a sling. For a fractured humerus place the collar and cuff under the patient's clothes.

Requirements:
  Collar and cuff bandage
  Safety pin

Application:
1 Allow the patient to place the hand across the chest.
2 Measure the appropriate amount of bandage required by looping the bandage around the wrist (Figure 16a) over the shoulder and back to the wrist (Figure 16b).
3 Cut at the appropriate length.
4 Place a safety pin in the bandage above the wrist (Figure 16c).

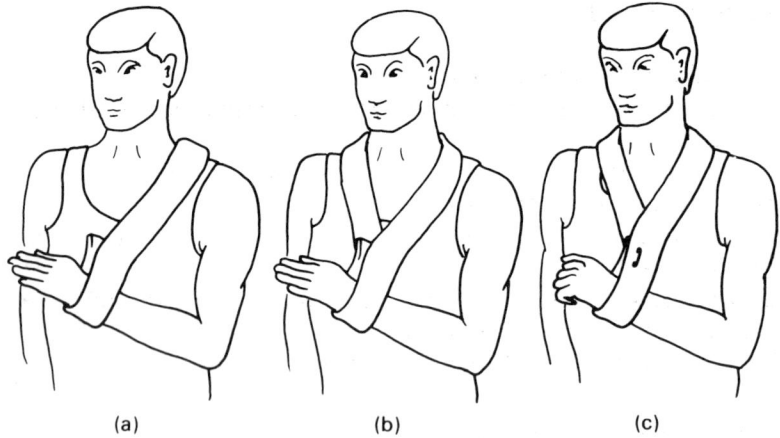

Figure 16 Application of a collar and cuff sling: measure the length of bandage required from the wrist (a) over the shoulder and back to the wrist (b). After cutting the bandage to the appropriate length, hold the sling in place using a safety pin (c).

Instructions for the patient:
1 Keep the arm in the bandage at all times except to dress.
2 Return to the fracture clinic for an appointment.

This collar and cuff must **not** be applied to patients who have injured their wrist.

Robert Jones Bandage. A Robert Jones bandage is applied to immobilize a limb after a non-fracture injury.

Requirements:
  Stockinette
  Brown cotton wool
  Domette bandage
  Crepe bandage, 15 cm

Application:
1 Remove clothing from the limb.
2 Position the leg in a slightly flexed position.
3 Apply the stockinette from the ankle to the groin (Figure 17a).
4 Wrap the brown cotton wool from the ankle to the groin over the stockinette (Figure 17b). Alternate the brown cotton wool with the domette in 3 layers (Figure 17c).
5 Wrap the crepe bandage over the wool and domette fairly firmly (Figure 17d).

Instructions for the patient:
1 The bandage is applied to prevent bending of the affected joint.
2 The bandage is to remain in place for 7 days or until an appointment at the fracture clinic.
3 When sitting, keep the leg elevated with the ankle above the height of the knee.
4 Crutches or a stick will be supplied depending on whether the limb can bear weight or not.
5 Tighten the crepe bandage as required by reapplying.

Sling. A sling can be applied for several reasons:
  To provide rest for a limb, e.g., a sprain.
  To give support, e.g., an arm in plaster of Paris.
  To reduce swelling and relieve pain, e.g., a high sling for a septic finger.

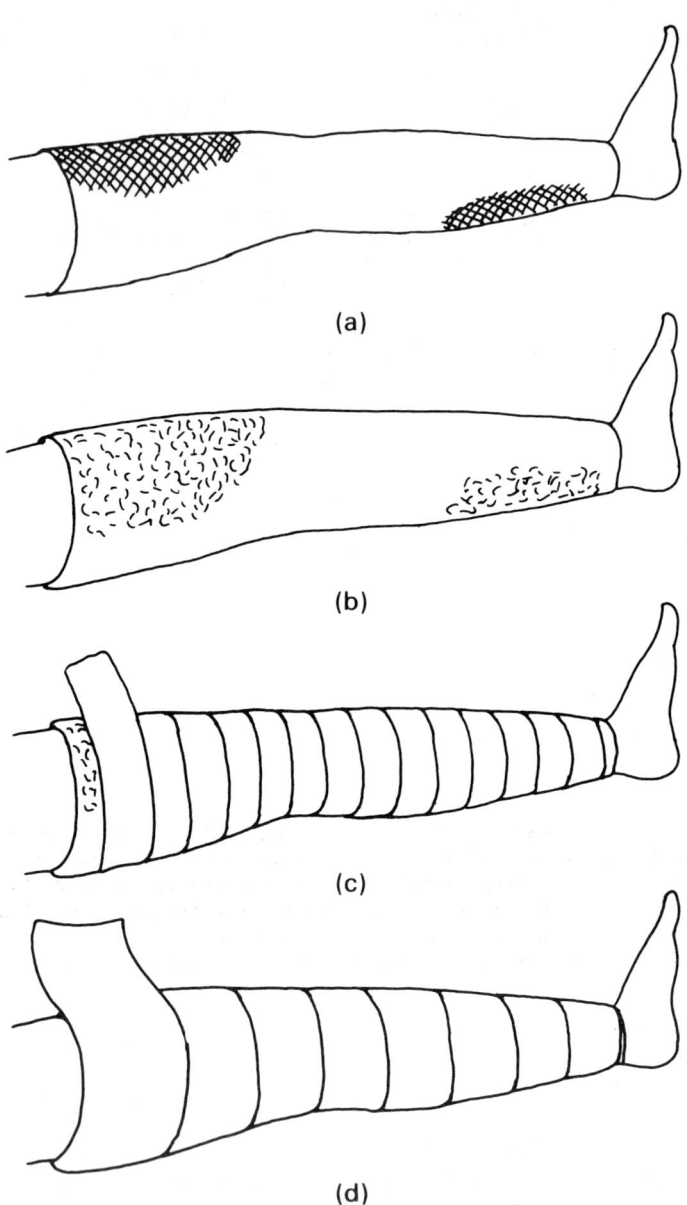

Figure 17 Application of a Robert Jones bandage: stockinette is applied from the ankle to the groin (a), and then wrapped in brown cotton wool (b), alternating with domette (c). Finally a crepe bandage is wrapped over the wool and domette (d).

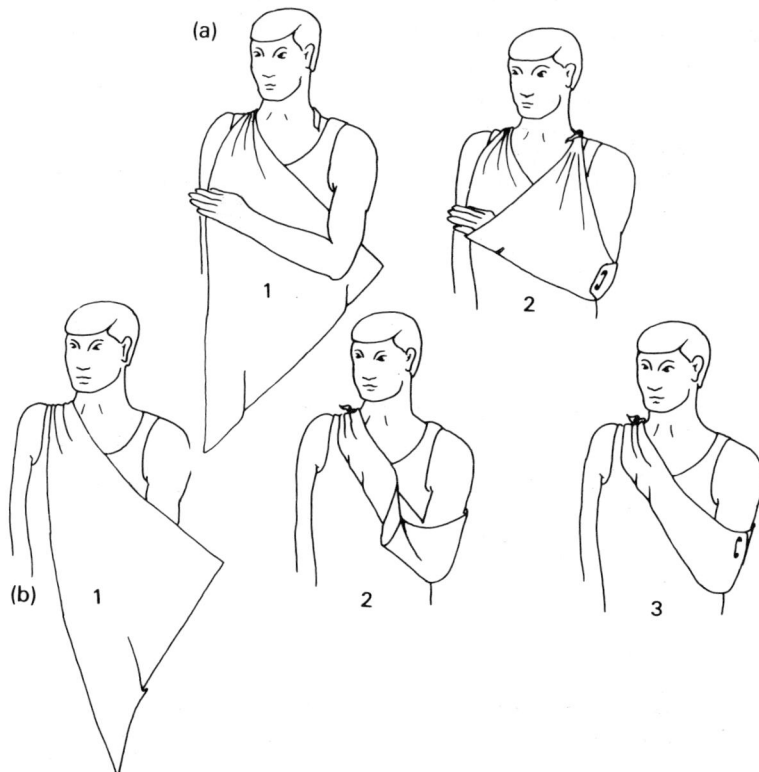

Figure 18 Application of a sling: with a low sling (a), the upper part of the sling is placed under the injured arm and over that shoulder (1). The lower point of the sling is placed over the affected shoulder around the arm and tied (2). With a high sling (b), the upper part of the sling is placed over the injured arm (1) and the lower point is placed under the elbow and behind the shoulder to be tied over the unaffected shoulder (2). The sling is secured with a safety pin (3).

Requirements:
  Sling
  Safety pin

Application of a low sling:
1 Stand and face the patient, holding the triangular corner of the sling against the affected elbow.
2 Place the upper part of the sling against the patient's chest and over the unaffected shoulder (Figure 18a (1)).
3 Allow the patient to place his or her arm up across the chest as high as possible.

Minor Injuries

4   Take the lower point of the sling up over the affected shoulder around the arm and tie a knot over the affected shoulder (Figure 18a (2)).

Application of a high sling:
1   Stand and face the patient, holding the sling against the patient as mentioned previously. However this time allow the patient to place the affected arm up towards the opposite shoulder under the sling (Figure 18b (1)).
2   Take the lower corner of the sling and put it under the elbow of the affected arm and up behind the shoulder to meet the other end of the sling, and knot over the unaffected shoulder (Figure 18b (2)).
3   Secure the sling with a safety pin as shown in Figure 18b (3).

Instructions for the patient:
1   The sling is applied to support the arm, and prevent any swelling.
2   When the arm is out of the sling it should be elevated on pillows.

Support Aids

Walking Stick

Instructions for the patient using a walking stick:
1   Stand up straight when the nurse gives you the walking stick so that the stick can be at the level of the top of your hip bone.
2   The hand in which to hold the stick will vary according to capabilities or other injuries. Opinions of departments may differ, but the best instruction would seem to be for the stick to be used in the hand of the affected side.
3   The stick should be moved forward and positioned on the floor just under one pace in front.
4   Lean on the stick and move the affected leg forward so that it is alongside the stick.
5   Still leaning on the stick, move the other leg forward and slightly ahead of the stick. Weight can then be transferred to the unaffected leg while the walking stick is again moved forward.

Points to remember:
The patient must not move the stick too far forward, thereby outstepping himself or herself.

Ensure that the walking stick is the correct height so that the patient does not have to stoop to use it.
Ensure that the walking stick has a rubber non slip end on it.
Ask the patient to return the stick to the department, when no longer needed, so that it can be used for other patients.
If the department keeps a record of equipment lent to patients, make sure that the patient signs for the walking stick.

Crutches

When fitting the patient for crutches make sure that the crutches are of the correct size. The size can be adjusted by the nuts and bolts on the crutches. To ascertain the correct size the patient must be standing upright and looking ahead. Remember, the reason for the crutches is to help the patient move without putting weight on the injured leg. Do not keep the patient standing too long at this stage and check that weight is not being put on to the injured leg.

With the patient standing upright place the crutches under his or her arms and measure to within two fingers width of the axilla (Figure 19). If this distance is kept between the crutches and the patient's axillae then there will be no risk of damage to the brachial nerve to the arms.

Allow the patient to sit while the nuts and bolts on the crutches are adjusted to the correct length. When this is done the patient must stand again so that the hand grips can be adjusted. With the patient standing upright and two fingers width between the top of the crutches and the axillae, the patient's hands should reach the hand grips with the elbows slightly flexed. Allow the patient to sit while these are being adjusted.

Instructions for the patient using crutches:
1 Stand correctly: up straight, head and eyes facing forward.
2 Position the crutches to be 10 cm in front and 10 cm to the side of the feet making a triangle.
3 Do not put any weight on the injured leg. The palms of the hands should grip the hand grips and the elbows should be slightly bent.
4 Keep shoulders and back straight. Do not bend to the crutches.

Minor Injuries

5 Lean the top of the crutches towards the chest and hold the upper arms against them. Do **not** lean the armpits on the crutches as this could cause serious injury to the nerve in the arm.

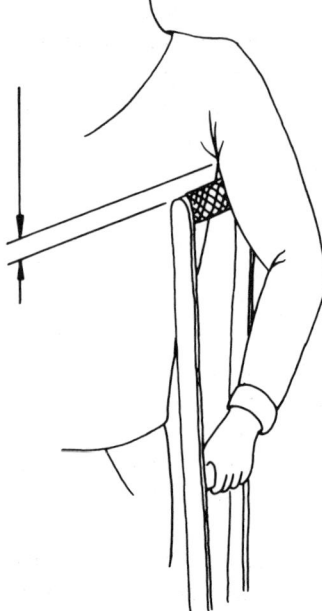

Figure 19 Correct method to hold a crutch. **Note** the arrows indicating that the width of two fingers must be maintained between the axilla and the crutch.

6 Start walking with the crutches by putting all the body weight on the good leg and moving both crutches forward about 30–45 cm and placing them firmly on the floor.
7 Transfer the weight to the crutches by leaning on the hands and swinging the body and legs forward until they are level with the crutches.
8 Remember to put the unaffected leg on the floor and move again.

Points for the patient to remember:
Do not lean the armpits on the crutches.
If arm pads or cushions are placed on the top of the crutches then the height of the crutches must be re-adjusted.
Re-adjust the height of the crutches if the height of the shoes is changed.
Each day examine the nuts and bolts on the crutches and tighten them if necessary.

Check the rubber end tips of the crutches weekly for wear and replace them as necessary.
Do not use crutches in socked feet or with open-toe shoes, but use firm strong shoes.
Beware of any objects on the floor which may cause a fall.
Return the crutches to the department when no longer needed.

These instructions may be given to the patient verbally or in writing. Make sure that the patient has practised and is able to use the crutches before leaving the department.

EPISTAXIS

Epistaxis (bleeding from the nose) a condition frequently encountered in the department, can be distressing for the patient.

The cause of a nose bleed can be undetermined though it can result from direct trauma, and generally resolves itself fairly quickly. It can also be caused by nasal infections or poking at the nostrils. It is often associated with hypertension and may be a safety release valve as the small capillaries in the nose break and blood is released.

As nose bleed can occur in a patient with hypertension it is vital that the blood pressure and pulse are recorded when the patient reaches the department. Blood loss can result in a low blood pressure and a rapid pulse but usually, although a patient with a nose bleed appears to be losing a tremendous amount of blood, it is not enough to cause the clinical condition of shock. A loss of between 15 % and 20 % of blood volume is needed for shock to manifest itself. In an adult with 5–6 litres of blood this would mean a loss of approximately 1500 ml of blood (equivalent to the average daily urine output or 3 fluid pints). It is not the clinical condition of shock which is usually dealt with but the anxiety and distress of the patient.

Patient Care

Sit the patient in an upright position and set your priorities:
Make sure that the patient has a **clear airway** and is not swallowing blood. Have the patient lean his or her head slightly forward. Ensure that the patient is provided with a bowl and tissues at this time.
Check the patient's **breathing** and provide reassurance.

Minor Injuries

Treatment

Control the bleeding if possible by:
1 Pinching the bridge of the patient's nose firmly and instructing the patient to breathe through the mouth
2 Placing an ice pack across the patient's nose.

Medical Intervention

Cautery. If neither treatment 1 or 2 is successful, inform the doctor who will examine the nostrils to see if the bleeding point can be located and cauterised.

Nasal packs. The doctor may decide to pack the nostrils with suitable material. For inserting nasal packs the equipment required will include:
  Tilley's nasal forceps
  Kidney dish
  Gallipot
  Ribbon gauze, 0.75 cm
The doctor may insert one of the following packs:
  Bismuth and iodoform paste — May be left in place for a week.
  Bismuth and glycerine — May be left in place for 48 hours.
  Petroleum jelly gauze — May be left in place for 48 hours.
With the latter two packs, the patient may receive antibiotics. If nasal packs are inserted the patient may be admitted to hospital. However, if the patient is sent home, he or she **must** be instructed to return to the Ear, Nose and Throat Clinic for the packs to be removed in 2 to 3 days.
  Be sure to advise the patient that, as breathing will be through the mouth only, the mouth will become dry and frequent mouth washes will alleviate discomfort.

Surgery. If bleeding is not controlled by cautery or packing then the patient may be admitted for surgery for the bleeding vessel to be tied off.
If the patient is admitted be sure that the next of kin is notified.

Instructions for the Patient

If the patient is treated in the department and then discharged he or she must be advised not to do anything which may aggravate the bleeding again and must avoid:
- Dry atmospheres
- Bending forward
- Sneezing or poking the nose
- Anything which may lead to a rise in blood pressure such as:
  - Excessive exercise
  - Emotional upsets
  - Constipation

The patient should be told to gently blow the nose only when absolutely necessary and report back to the doctor if bleeding recurs.

Continual Discharge

As mentioned before, nasal bleeding due to a traumatic incident usually resolves quickly and does not produce a continual discharge. Ensure that nasal bleeding following a traumatic incident is purely bleeding from the nostrils.

Continual discharge (*rhinorrhoea*) of a serosanguineous looking fluid may be cerebrospinal fluid indicating that the patient has a fractured base of skull. If the fluid when tested contains glucose and protein then it is cerebrospinal fluid (see Chapter 8).

EYE INJURY

The eye is a very delicate structure (Figure 20) and injury to the eye is very worrying for the patient. Many eye injuries can be easily treated in an accident and emergency department and the patient discharged home with very little after effects. However, eye conditions must be handled skilfully to prevent further complications.

Chemicals in the Eye

If a patient has splashed any chemical substance in the eye it will cause burning.

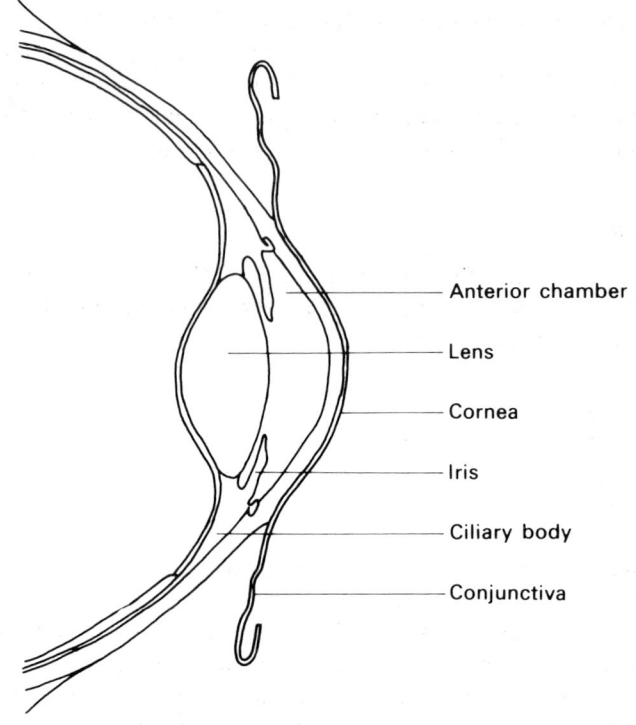

Figure 20 Cross section of the eye showing the structures that may be damaged by small objects in the eye.

First Aid Measures

Treatment **must** commence immediately in the first aid situation to prevent the burning continuing. To do this the chemical must be washed out of the eye by gentle irrigation with sterile water or tap water.

Remember that the patient will be experiencing a lot of pain from the burning in the eye and may be unable to co-operate and hold the eye open. If this is the case then the nurse needs to hold the patient's eye open with the thumb and finger or lid retractors in order to continue the irrigation. The patient may be in a sitting position with the head tilted backwards or may be lying down for this procedure.

Do not put the water directly onto the eye as the coldness will startle the patient. Instead drop a little water onto the patient's face, i.e., on the cheek, before moving the water towards the inner corner of the eye. As the patient is unable to see what is happening give plenty of warning while performing this procedure. The irrigation should be continued until the patient does not feel any burning in the eye. The patient must then be transported to the accident and emergency department.

Treatment

If the procedure for the irrigation of the eye has not been completed in the first aid situation then this treatment must be carried out in the department.

Equipment needed:
  Protection for the patient
  Kidney dish to be held beside the eye to catch the irrigating fluid
  Utensil to hold the irrigating fluid — an undine
  Irrigating fluid, i.e., tepid sterile water

The patient may be in a sitting position with the head tilted backwards or may be lying down for this procedure.

Remember to reassure the patient and to warn against rubbing the eye or eyes. Due to the fact that the eye is such a delicate organ the doctor should be informed so that the patient can be seen as soon as possible, especially in the case of an object in the eye.

Material in the Eye

The patient with material in the eye **must** be advised not to rub the eye but to keep it shut. It is best to advise the patient to keep both eyes shut as the movement of one eye also leads to the movement of the other. The patient may have both eyes padded to prevent eye movement. Be sure to speak to and reassure the patient because by now there may be a double anxiety. Firstly, worry about damage to the eye and secondly, a worry about what is going on around them.

Make sure that the patient is sitting securely in an area where the doctor can examine the eye. Some departments have rooms with equipment for eye examinations whilst others may send the patient to the eye clinic for treatment.

Treatment

The treatment of a patient with material in the eye depends on the amount, size, type and location of the substance.

Amount and Size. If there are one or two larger pieces the doctor may be able to remove these with a sterile cotton wool bud.

Type. If the object is metal then a magnet can be used to remove it. However, if there is a lot of dust or material in the eye which is resting on the cornea then the doctor may order an eye irrigation.

Location. Any material in the eye which is resting on the cornea may be removed by the doctor or by irrigation. However, if the object has embedded itself in the cornea and possibly penetrated to the lens or other parts of the eye, then this must be removed by a surgical procedure. This will necessitate the patient's admission to hospital for surgery and for further observation following surgery.

Following removal of the object or objects from above the cornea the doctor will then examine the eye to ensure that no damage is present. Objects in the eye can scrape the cornea and cause a *corneal abrasion.* It may be possible to see the abrasion on examination or the doctor may instil a fluorescent dye which will show the abrasion as a yellow discolouration.

The treatment for a corneal abrasion is to rest the eye so the patient is advised to wear an eye pad for several days. Also to prevent any infection the patient is instructed to instil antibiotic drops in the eye, such as Chloramphenicol, twice a day. As a prophylactic measure most patients who have been treated for objects in the eye are given a 5-day course of antibiotic eye drops.

Discharging the Patient

When a patient is discharged from the department ensure that the patient, relative or friend knows how to instill the eye drops and has these instructions:
1   Open the eye by holding upper lid and lower lid with first and second finger.

2 Tilt head back and look towards ceiling.
3 Having first removed cap from bottle lift bottle to above eye where it can be seen.
4 Invert bottle and drop one eye drop between lower lid and eye ball (Figure 21).

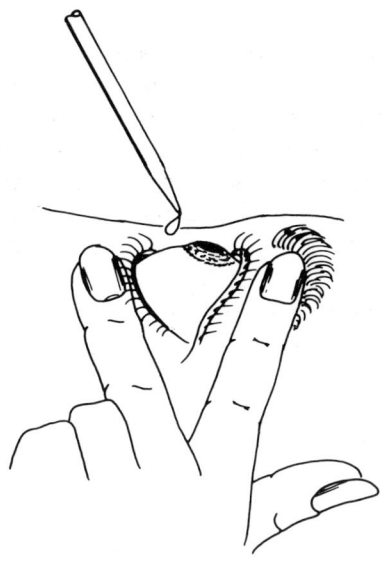

Figure 21 Application of eye drops. **Note** the placing of the fingers to maintain the position of the upper and lower eye lids to allow insertion of the drops under the lower lid.

5 Close eye, wipe away excess from eyelashes.
6 Replace eye pad with eye closed. If an eye pad is not being worn then the patient can open the eye and blink several times to distribute the antibiotic.

Also ensure that the patient:
  Can obtain the prescribed eye drops.
  Has analgesia if necessary.
  Is accompanied if discharged wearing an eye pad.
Find out from the doctor when the patient may return to work. If the eye injury means time off work then ensure that the patient has a sick note.
If a patient wearing an eye pad lives alone, make sure that he or she can manage with cooking, eating, washing etc.
The patient wearing an eye pad should **not** drive a car, operate machinery, drink alcohol, work at any height, play sports, or work in a furnace.

Wearing an eye pad, until a patient is used to it, can create misconception of distance, so the patient must be warned of this hazard. Even if the patient goes home without an eye patch he or she must be warned of the possibility of poor vision for a time, especially if the doctor has administered a mydriatic eye drop to enable clearer vision of the eye. A *mydriatic* drug has the same effect on the pupil of the eye as does the sympathetic nervous system when it is stimulated. That is, it dilates the pupil of the

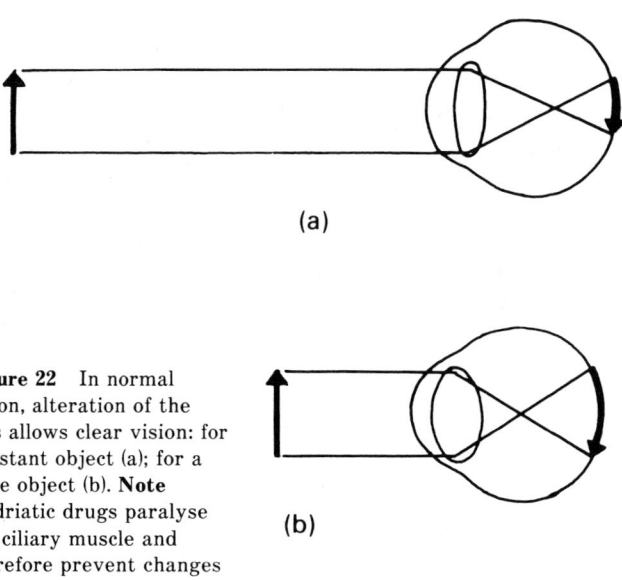

Figure 22 In normal vision, alteration of the lens allows clear vision: for a distant object (a); for a close object (b). **Note** mydriatic drugs paralyse the ciliary muscle and therefore prevent changes in lens shape and pupil size in response to light.

eye which means that the refraction of light is altered. The adaptation of the pupil aperture and the shape of the lens allows the eye to accommodate for vision (Figure 22). However, after a mydriatic drug such as Mydriacyl has been administered the pupil is unable to constrict for a period of 3 hours, so that the image is not accurately focused on the retina to allow clear vision. If atropine eye drops are administered it may be several days before the pupil is able to constrict normally.

REVISION OBJECTIVES

1 Name and describe the type of minor injuries patients may sustain and the methods of patient care and treatment for each injury.
2 Describe the wound healing process.
3 Explain the blood-clotting mechanism.
4 Describe the inflammatory reaction.
5 Identify the stages of anaesthesia.
6 Describe the care of a patient undergoing a general anaesthetic within the department.
7 Describe aseptic techniques and the care of minor injuries.
8 Elaborate on the importance and the administration of tetanus toxoid.
9 Demonstrate the application of supportive bandages.
10 Instruct a patient requiring aids for walking.
11 Describe the care of a patient following an epistaxis.
12 Describe the care of a patient following an eye injury.
13 Counsel patients prior to discharge on the care of minor injuries sustained.

5
Cardiac Emergencies

THE HEART

The heart is composed of three separate layers of different tissue: the pericardium, the myocardium and the endothelium.

The outer layer is a fibrous coating known as the **pericardium**. It is composed of two layers:

The visceral layer covering the outside.

The parietal layer coating the heart.

The two layers have smooth surfaces which allow the heart to move freely without causing friction.

The middle layer is the heart muscle known as the **myocardium**. The heart muscle is described as being striated (striped in appearance). Like all muscle it is controlled by part of the nervous system. It is an involuntary control governed by both parts of the autonomic nervous system:

Parasympathetic system which functions via the vagus nerves (the tenth pair of cranial nerves) and decreases the force and the rate of the heart.

Sympathetic system which comes from the cervical sympathetic nerve ganglion and increases the force and rate of the heart.

Also the heart is unique as it has an innate beating action which means that the heart muscle can contract on its own. However these innate contractions are not able to produce a co-ordinated and sufficient heart beat to circulate blood around the body.

The inner layer known as the **endocardium** is composed of the same smooth epithelial cells which line the blood vessels.

CORONARY ARTERIES

The heart muscle receives its own blood supply via the coronary

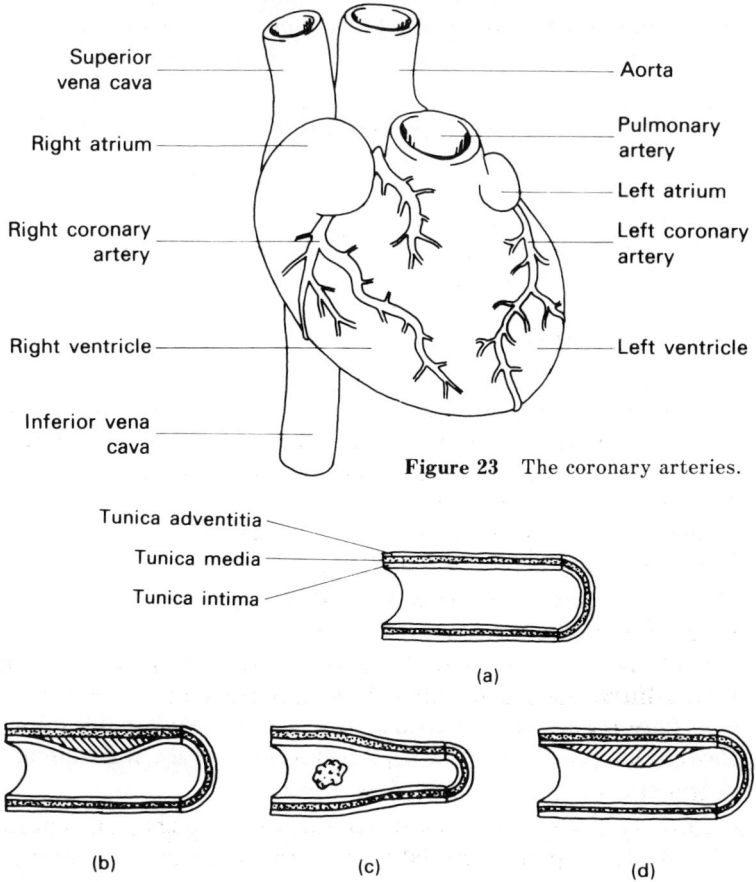

Figure 23 The coronary arteries.

Figure 24 The normal artery (a), and disorders within the arteries: atheroma (b); embolus (c); thrombosis (d).

arteries (Figure 23) which are the first arteries to divide from the aorta. What happens when these arteries become diseased depends on the area of heart tissue affected and the amount of blockage within the artery.

Causes of Blockage

Blockage within the arteries can be caused by the deposit of fatty plaques, an embolus or a thrombus (Figure 24).

The deposit of **fatty plaques** within the artery *(atheroma)* causes constriction and narrowing of the lumen of the artery (Figure 24b).

An **embolus** is a fragment of a blood clot. It travels in the blood stream until it becomes lodged in a small artery anywhere in the body (commonly occurring in the pulmonary circulation and the coronary circulation) and causes complete obstruction of the artery (Figure 24c).

A **thrombus** is the formation by gradual deposits of substances within an artery or vein until there is either partial or complete blockage caused by the deposits or an embolus at the site (Figure 24d).

Arterial Disorders

Disorders within the arteries of the heart are known as angina or myocardial infarction.

Angina

Angina occurs when the blood vessels have narrowed sufficiently to impede, at times, the blood flow to the heart muscle. The size of the lumen of the blood vessels becomes smaller but cigarette smoking can also contribute to this by causing general vasoconstriction thereby actually making the artery narrower from without. This results in a restriction of the blood flow to the area of heart muscle concerned, especially in times of increased circulatory demand such as walking and exercising.

Signs and Symptoms. In angina the onset will have been sudden but connected with some form of exertion. The pain may have lasted for only a few minutes because the patient will have stopped the exertion and rested, so allowing the heart muscle to obtain a sufficient blood supply. The patient will state that the pain was sharp and either located in the left side of the chest only or in the left side of the chest and radiating down the left arm. The pain might have made the patient feel nauseated and even produced vomiting or caused profuse sweating *(diaphoresis)*. Other associated symptoms are dizziness, palpitations and shortness of breath.

Myocardial Infarction

Myocardial infarction or coronary thrombosis is a complete blockage in any part of the coronary arteries caused by either a thrombus or an embolus on top of a thrombus. This means, as the word suggests, that the heart muscle is affected and there is irreparable damage to the area of heart muscle without a blood supply due to the complete blockage of the artery.

Signs and Symptoms. In the case of a myocardial infarction the patient might appear in much the same condition as the patient with angina but there are some very important differences. The patient with a myocardial infarction has suffered permanent damage to some part of the heart muscle. The severity of the patient's symptoms will depend on the extent and the area of the heart muscle affected.

Characteristically, the patient may complain of a gripping chest pain as if there is a tight belt around the chest; this pain may also extend down the left arm or up into the jaw. The pain is continual and indefinite as nothing the patient can do seems to relieve it. The pain is not related to exercise and can come on at any time even during the night.

The patient's general condition is liable to be one of shock, although patients are known to present with no signs of shock and only a mild complaint of a pain like indigestion. If the patient is in a condition of shock this will mean that there is some change in the patient's heart function due to heart damage or the severity of the pain. In either case the patient will appear:
Pale
Diaphoretic
Cold to touch
Anxious and restless

These factors have been listed in the order in which the signs are observed, indicating that urgent notice **must** be taken of the patient and the condition dealt with immediately. During observation of the patient in shock, the pulse and blood pressure will be noted:

The **pulse** is rapid and thready. The patient can have a tachycardia of over 120 beats per minute.

The **blood pressure** is low (hypotensive). It may even be impossible to record a blood pressure using a sphygmomanometer in which case the pressure may be estimated by palpation of the radial pulse. This will only give the systolic pressure of the heart.

The patient may also complain of nausea and vomiting, palpitations, dizziness and shortness of breath or even dyspnoea (difficulty in breathing).

Immediate Treatment

Immediate treatment means immediate in two senses. The patient must be seen by the doctor and the patient's condition must be assessed.

Examination by a Doctor

Any patient with chest pain **must** be seen immediately by the doctor. This may mean that this patient will be seen before some patients who have been waiting longer with other complaints. This factor you must appreciate may cause problems. Other patients may have seen this patient, complaining of chest pain, walk into the hospital looking relatively well and note that this person is seen immediately by the nurse and doctor for no obvious reason.

No complaint of chest pain should be taken lightly until examination reveals otherwise.

Patient Assessment

First assess the patient's general condition and then take a careful history from the patient.

General Condition. Assess the patient's condition for immediate care:
Check that the **airway is patent.**
If the airway is clear, check that **breathing is adequate.** Observe especially for any difficulty in breathing or any cyanosis. Treat the condition according to the symptoms:
1 Sit the patient upright or in a semirecumbent position to enable easier breathing. Remember to record the blood pressure as a patient with severe hypotension may need to be nursed in a semirecumbent position not upright. Sitting upright may lower the blood pressure and take blood away from the brain.
2 Loosen any tight clothing especially around the neck, chest or abdomen.
3 Prepare to administer oxygen by facial mask.

Observe the function of the cardiovascular system:
1 Record the blood pressure.
2 Take and record the pulse either as a radial pulse or as a recording of the apex beat of the heart.

3 Prepare an intravenous infusion for the administration of drugs and fluids.

During the assessment of the patient any care or treatment which is essential to maintain the patient's life must be carried out (see Chapter 3).

Brief History. If the patient's condition is fairly stable then the nurse can continue the assessment by obtaining a brief history from the patient to ascertain the condition. This can be done by asking questions related to the signs and symptoms:
1 What is the pain like?
2 When did you first notice the pain?
3 Can you do anything to relieve the pain?
4 Where is the pain located? Does the pain move?
5 Have you had the pain before? If the answer is yes, what happened on that occasion?

Ask the patient to take a deep breath if at all possible. Observe whether this is aggravating the pain or not. If the patient has angina then the deep breath may even help the pain. If the patient has a myocardial infarction the deep breath will not affect the pain.

The patient may have difficulty in taking a deep breath due to the severity of the pain. If the patient has extreme difficulty and increasing pain on taking a deep breath then this might indicate that the patient has a respiratory problem rather than a heart complaint (see Chapter 6).

Diagnostic Tests

A brief history can help towards a diagnosis but it will take the doctor's examination and the results of some or all of the following tests to definitely confirm the condition. These tests, an electrocardiogram (ECG) and blood-specimen assays, can either individually or in combination confirm that a patient has suffered a myocardial infarction. There may be changes on the ECG when a patient suffers from angina but as there is no permanent damage to the heart muscle the blood tests remain unchanged.

ECG

An ECG is a recording of the conduction of the electrical

impulses in the heart resulting in the action of heart muscle (see p.116). At present the taking and recording of an ECG is not a nursing responsibility. However nurses may assist in preparing the patient for the test.

Blood Specimens

Blood specimens are taken to analyse the serum enzymes, estimate the number of leucocytes and the erythrocyte sedimentation rate.

Serum Enzymes. An enzyme is a substance produced by living cells to promote specific chemical changes. All enzymes are known to be proteins and they are very susceptible to changes in acidity and changes in temperature. When the heart muscle is damaged enzymes are released into the bloodstream and their level can be measured. The changes are not always immediate so the test is repeated for several days and until the results are within normal limits.

The enzymes which are produced are: glutamic oxaloacetic transaminase (SGOT) or aspartate transaminase (ASPT) — this change usually occurs quite quickly and may last for several days: and lactic dehydrogenase (LDH) or hydroxybutyrate dehydrogenase (HBD) — this change is more gradual and may remain altered for several weeks.

Leucocyte Count. Due to the damage of the heart tissue the leucocyte (white cell) count is raised for several days (normal 4000–10 000 mm^{-3}).

Erythrocyte Sedimentation Rate. An increase in the erythrocyte sedimentation rate (ESR) can indicate an increase in fibrinogen, a plasma protein which is present to initiate clotting by converting to fibrin after bleeding has occurred. Due to the changes in the myocardium of the heart and the death (necrosis) of the muscle the erythrocyte sedimentation rate is often raised following a myocardial infarction and it can remain raised for several days.

Administration of Drugs

Drugs may be given to alleviate pain and anxiety, correct the strength and rhythm of the heart's action or assist respiration.

Alleviate Pain and Anxiety. The drug to alleviate pain and anxiety is morphine or diamorphine. This is administered intramuscularly at a dose of 5-15 mg immediately and then at 4-6 hourly intervals as necessary. This is a controlled drug and has several effects. It tranquillizes which helps to relieve the anxiety but can also make the patient euphoric. Adverse effects of the drug can result in respiratory depression, hypotension, nausea and vomiting. The main problem for the patient following a myocardial infarction is the nausea and vomiting caused by morphine and the patient's general condition. To alleviate this an antiemetic is usually given with the morphine — cyclizine hydrochloride, 50 mg given intramuscularly.

For angina, glyceryl trinitrate tablets (0.5-1 mg) may be given sublingually as desired or by mouth as sustained-release tablets (2.6-6.4 mg), 2-3 times a day. The tablets act as vasodilators and dilate the coronary arteries and other arteries of the body which is why a patient may complain of a headache or look flushed.

Correct Heart Action. The heart action may have been altered in strength, rate and rhythm. Digoxin has three well known actions it slows, strengthens and steadies the heart. For very rapid control digoxin may be given intravenously in a dose from 0.75-1.25 mg. It is important to have the patient connected to an ECG machine if the drug is administered in this way so there is a complete picture of the heart action. Digoxin can also be given intramuscularly as Lanoxin 250 mg ml^{-1}. Digoxin is the drug of choice when a patient has tachycardia.

When the patient has received damage to the heart which has resulted in a slow heart action *(bradycardia)* then atropine 0.3 - 1 mg may be given intravenously.

Both the above mentioned drugs alter the rate of the heart and also the strength, allowing for an adequate circulation.

If the heart rhythm has been disturbed and there are irregular heart actions then lignocaine hydrochloride may be given. A bolus of lignocaine hydrochloride may be given intravenously followed by an infusion containing lignocaine hydrochloride. The lignocaine hydrochloride infusion should be continued for 36 hours. Other drugs that also treat arrhythmias are procainamide hydrochloride (Pronestyl) and practolol (Eraldin).

Assist Respiration. Aminophylline may be given to aid the respiratory function. It is given slowly by intravenous injection 250–500 mg. It relaxes smooth muscle and dilates bronchi, increases the heart rate, strengthens the heart beat and has a diuretic action.

If it is confirmed that the patient has had a myocardial infarction then the patient will require admission to hospital so the nearest relative must be informed. In the case of angina the patient may be admitted to hospital for rest and further investigations.

HEART MUSCLE

Although the heart muscle has an innate beating action the muscle is co-ordinated into effective action by nerve impulses originating from the sinoatrial node in the right atrium of the heart (Figure 25).

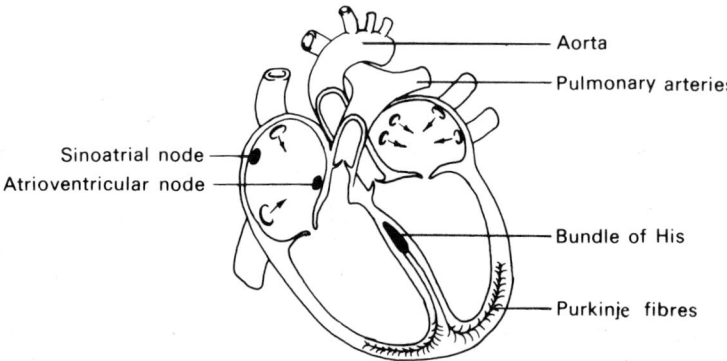

Figure 25 The conduction mechanism of the heart.

Sinoatrial Node

The sinoatrial node is a specialized neuromuscular tissue found at the junction of the superior vena cava and the right atrium. The node is stimulated by the right branch of the vagus nerve.

The sinoatrial node initiates heart action by sending impulses across and down the atria (both left and right atrium) to the tissue known as the atrioventricular node. These impulses cause the atria to contract together (Figure 26a). Once the impulses have passed through the atria they leave the atrioventricular node and arrive in the septum (the partition between the left and right ventricle), an area of specialized tissue known as the bundle of His. From the bundle of His the impulses are conducted

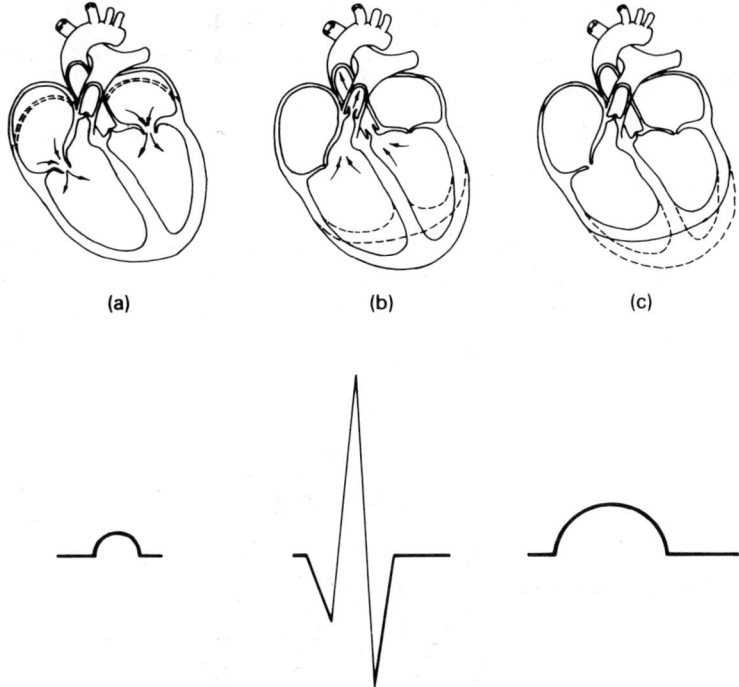

Figure 26 Heart action *(hatched lines)* and related movement of blood (arrows) through the heart in sequence, related to an electrocardiogram: as the atria contract (a), blood is forced into the ventricles; the ventricles contract and blood is pumped into the pulmonary artery and the aorta (b); the ventricles relax and return to their original size (c).

around the base of the ventricles along fibres known as the Purkinje fibres. The ventricles of the heart are then stimulated to contract simultaneously (Figure 26b). The ventricles then relax and return to their original size (Figure 26c).

It is these actions of the heart which are demonstrated on the electrocardiogram (Figure 26).

The Electrocardiogram

A normal heart rhythm is known as a sinus rhythm. This means the heart beat is being initiated and controlled by the sinoatrial node. To record the electrical changes that take place in the heart as a result of its beat, electrodes from the electrocardiograph machine are connected to the patient. At present there are two types of electrodes which need to be attached to the patient (Figure 27a and c) to produce an electrocardiogram (ECG) — a tracing of the heart's action. For additional recordings, chest leads can also be used (Figure 27b). On reading an ECG a normal sinus rhythm should appear and each significant pulse is denoted by a letter (Figure 28).

The **P wave** denotes the contraction of the atria after the impulse has spread from the sinoatrial node.

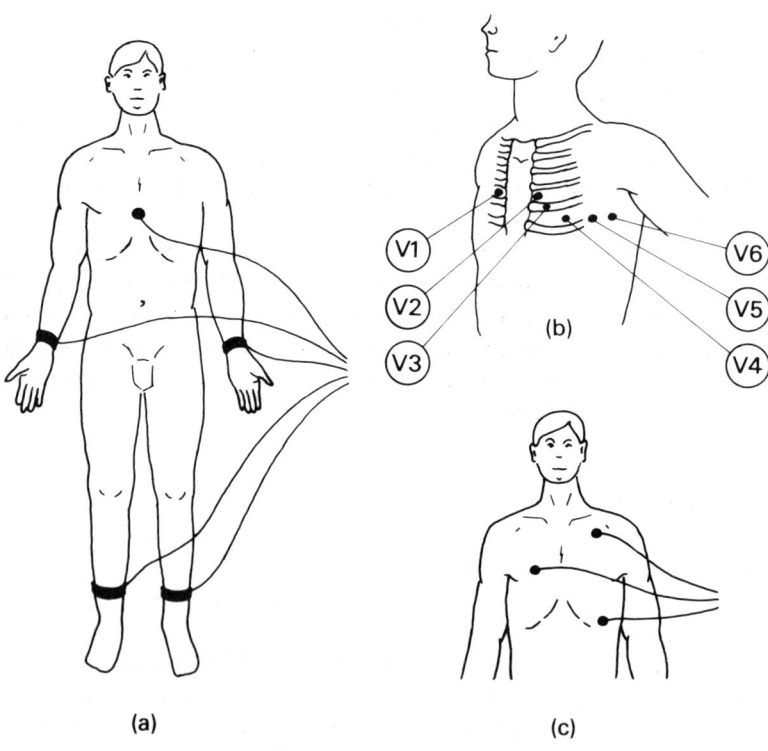

Figure 27 Heart monitoring: position of electrodes for recording an electrocardiogram (a); position of chest leads, V1 to V6, for additional recording of heart action (b); position of electrodes for continuous monitoring (c).

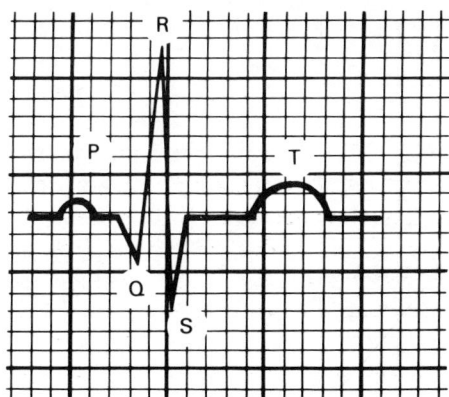

Figure 28 Sinus rhythm: a normal electrocardiogram recording as it appears on the recording paper. **Note** letters, PQRST, are related to specific heart activity.

The QRS impulses are known as the **QRS complex** as they all denote the contraction of both the ventricles. It is this impulse and movement of the ventricles which pumps the blood into the aorta and around the body.

The **T wave** is the recording as the ventricles relax back to their original shape ready to receive blood from the atria again.

The flat line following the T wave is a period of heart rest when there are no electrical changes or activity.

The PQRST action occurs about 72 times a minute in normal health.

At present the role of the trained nurse in the accident and emergency department has not extended to the responsibility of recording or reading an ECG. This requires the skill of a trained doctor. However in cases when a doctor needs assistance in recording an ECG, the nurse needs to be able to recognize certain heart changes.

ALTERATIONS IN HEART RHYTHM

Alterations in heart rhythm *(arrhythmias)* can involve the rate or the regularity as well as gross abnormalities of the heart beat.

Rate. The rate of the heart beat can be firstly recorded as a radial pulse beat or an apex heart beat and then demonstrated on an ECG tracing. The ECG paper is marked in time spaces. For the normal heart beat the PQRST tracing should occur within squares which would equal a heart beat of 72 a minute (Figure 29).

Cardiac Emergencies 117

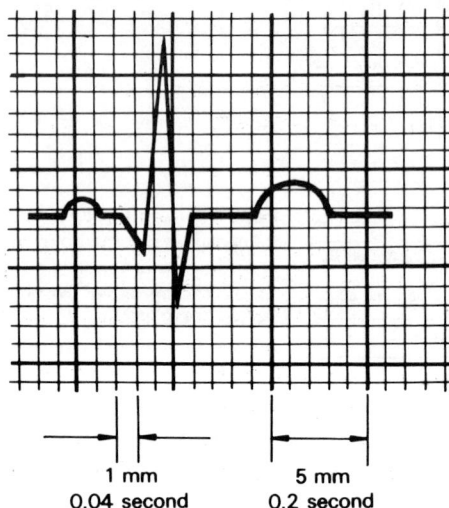

Figure 29 Electrocardiogram showing the normal time spacing.

Regularity. The regularity of the heart beat may have been first demonstrated by the recording of the radial pulse or the apex beat. However the regularity can also be shown on the ECG tracing by a regular, repeated pattern of the PQRST tracing. If this is not regular then the nurse should be able to tell how often the same pattern is repeated and what differences are occuring in a stated time.

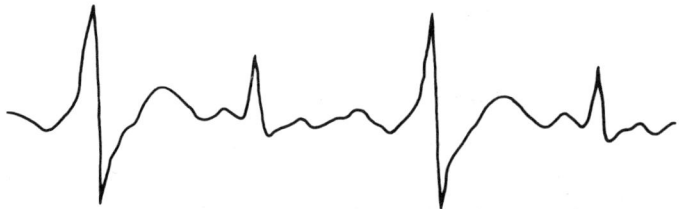

Figure 30 Ectopic beats, alternating with a normal heart beat.

In Figure 30, the tracing shows a patient who is having abnormal electrical impulses every other heart beat. The abnormal impulses are known as ectopic beats and if the patient's pulse rate is 104 beats per minute then in this example the abnormalities are occuring at the rate of 52 a minute. This would be a serious condition and the patient would require **urgent** treatment.

Gross Abnormalities. The nurse should be able to recognize the gross abnormalities of heart action as they are shown on the ECG.

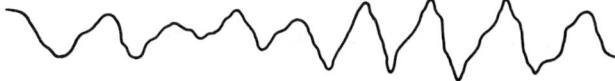

Figure 31 Ventricular fibrillation, an ineffective heart action.

Ventricular fibrillation is the result of multiple nerve impulses which result in the heart quivering like a jelly unable to contract adequately to pump blood around the body (Figure 31).

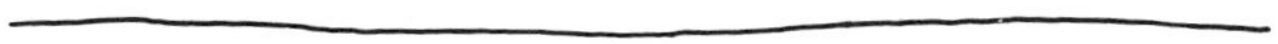

Figure 32 Cardiac asystole, no heart beat.

Cardiac asystole is when the heart is without a sinus rhythm. The heart has stopped beating; it is a cardiac arrest (Figure 32).

Both of these conditions, ventricular fibrillation and cardiac asystole, leave the patient without an adequate blood circulation, blood pressure or pulse and the patient requires **immediate** resuscitation. The treatment of cardiac arrhythmias depends on the resultant changes in heart action.

Atrial Fibrillation

Atrial fibrillation is when there are numerous nervous stimuli bombarding the atria and the muscle of the atria move in response, thereby producing over activity, and a rapid-beating atrium (Figure 33). The patient presents with complaints of

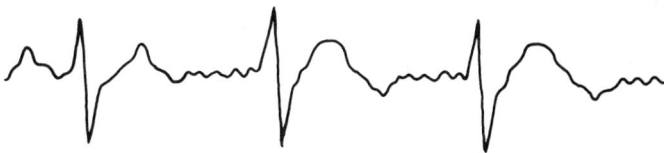

Figure 33 Atrial fibrillation, the normal 'P' wave is absent and is replaced by a quivering rapid atrial heart action.

weakness, nausea, pallor, dizziness and palpitations (when the patient is actually aware of the heart's beat). The patient may even be in a state of shock if the heart action is sufficiently interrupted.

The radial pulse beats are irregular and uneven in strength. This is because the ventricles are affected by the atria not pumping blood into them. Therefore, very little blood is pumped from the ventricles into the aorta on some beats with a resulting low pressure in the circulation. Also, the conduction of impulses through the heart is disturbed in the atria initially which affects the ventricles. This condition results in an apex heart beat that is at times more rapid than the radial pulse rate.

Treatment

Treatment can be by drug therapy or stimulation of the vagus nerve.

Drug therapy is given to slow and co-ordinate the action of the atrium. Digoxin can be used in this case.

Stimulation of the vagus nerve might revert the heart back to its normal sinoatrial control but must be carried out in the presence of a doctor. Vagal stimulation can be affected by putting pressure on one of the carotid sinuses by stroking the carotid artery, or by putting pressure over the eye balls.

Heart Block

Heart block results from some interference of the conduction of the nerve impulse at any point along the conduction pathways and the patient's ECG will be similar to Figure 34. Due to some nerve impulses not getting through the heart muscle, the patient will have a slow pulse rate *(bradycardia)*. The patient may present with no signs or symptoms except for the slow pulse rate which can be demonstrated on the ECG, or the patient may have a history of periods of sudden collapse when the heart has

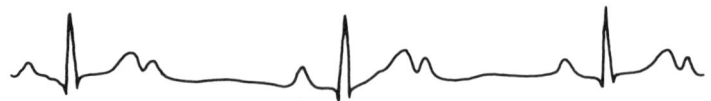

Figure 34 Heart block, the heart beat is slower.
Note the normal time interval.

stopped temporarily resulting in a lack of blood to the brain, e.g., Stokes-Adams syndrome.

Treatment

The treatment depends on the severity of the condition. There are several drugs to be given:
    Atropine 0.3–1 mg
    Isoprenaline 0.5–10 mg min^{-1}
In severe cases of heart block the patient may require a pacemaker to be inserted which will take over the conducting mechanism of the heart.

Ectopic Beats

The patient with irregular heart rhythms or abnormal or extra heart beats such as the ectopic beats will require stabilization of the heart before they develop the serious abnormality of ventricular fibrillation (see Figure 30 and 31).

Ectopic refers to an abnormal anatomical situation. In the heart it refers to an area of myocardium that is sending off abnormal electrical stimuli which result in abnormal action or contraction of the heart muscle.

Treatment

The drugs used in this treatment depend on the heart rate.
    Digoxin — to slow and steady the heart.
    Quinidine — to calm the ectopic activity.
    Lignocaine hydrochloride — to control the excitability of the heart.

Ventricular Fibrillation

The ECG of a patient with ventricular fibrillation shows total disturbance of the P wave (see Figure 31). Grossly abnormal arrhythmia, ventricular fibrillation and the situation of no heart action manifest themselves in the same way when you observe the patient and the treatment is to restore as soon as possible an adequate heart action.

Treatment

For treatment of inadequate heart action an electrical defibrillator may be used (Figure 35a). The defibrillator delivers an electrical shock to the patient in order to try and correct the abnormal activity. If the defibrillation has been effective then the patient's heart should return to the normal sinus rhythm.

Before use the defibrillator machine must be turned on and set at the correct electrical charge according to the doctor's instructions. The defibrillator paddles are then covered by an electrode jelly or an electrode pad to prevent the electric shock from burning the patient's skin. There are two electrodes that are positioned on the patient's chest, one over the apex of the heart and one on the sternum (Figure 35c).

The doctor will administer the electric shock (Figure 35b) but **remember** to stand clear of the patient and the bed to prevent receiving the shock yourself.

To observe the results of the defibrillation the patient must be connected to the ECG machine for regular monitoring.

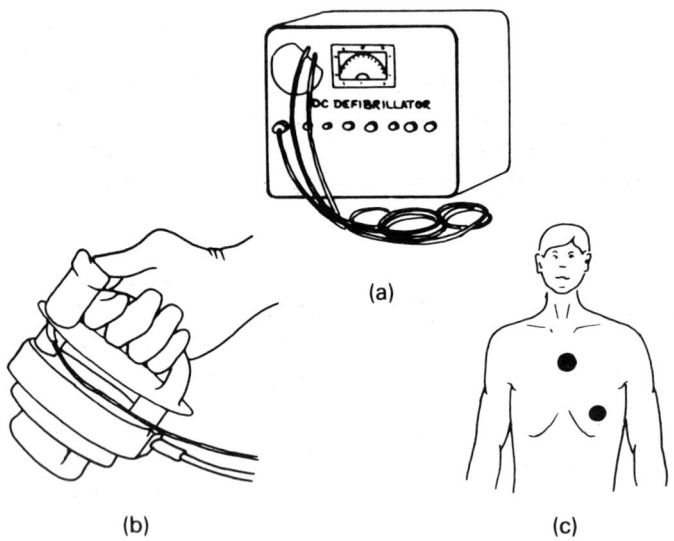

Figure 35 Electrical defibrillation: a defibrillator (a), the machine emits an electrical impulse to the patient and the amount of impulse must be set on the dial before use; one of the two defibrillator paddles (b), the thumb shows the position of the button which imparts the impulse; area on the patient where the corresponding defibrillator paddles are placed (c), one on the sternum, the other on the apex of the heart.

Cardiac Asystole

A cardiac asystole occurs when the heart has stopped beating and there is no sinus rhythm.

Treatment

To treat cardiac asystole the heart will be stimulated into action by external or internal massage (see Chapter 3) and by the action of drugs:
   Adrenaline
   Atropine

ACUTE LEFT VENTRICULAR FAILURE

Acute left ventricular failure involves the inability of the left ventricle to perform its function of receiving blood from the left atrium and pumping the blood through the aorta and around the body.

Normally, oxygenated blood is received from the lungs via the four pulmonary veins into the left atrium. From the left atrium blood is pushed through the mitral valve (biscuspid valve) into the left ventricle. Once the left ventricle has received the blood the mitral valve closes and as the ventricle contracts to pump, the aortic valve opens and blood is pushed into the aorta (Figure 36).

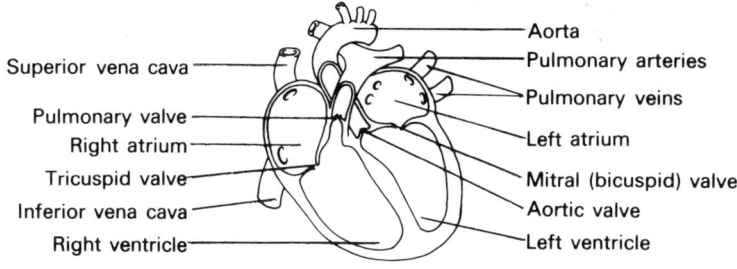

Figure 36 Structure of a normal heart.

In left ventricular failure several things can happen:
The ventricle cannot pump with enough force so that some blood remains within the ventricle.
The mitral valve does not close completely so some blood is

Cardiac Emergencies

forced by the pumping action of the left ventricle not only into the aorta but back into the left atrium.

The aortic valve does not close sufficiently after the ventricle has contracted to push blood into the aorta so that some blood returns into the left ventricle.

The result is that the left ventricle becomes distended with blood and so enlarges. The contraction of the heart muscle becomes weaker and the blood begins to accumulate not only in the left ventricle but in the left atrium and in the lungs (pulmonary circulation).

Causes

Failure of the left ventricle can be caused by disease or hypertension.

Disease can occur:

Within the left ventricle or to the muscle of the left ventricle.

Within the coronary arteries affecting the blood supply to the ventricles or the left ventricular muscle.

Within the valves which connect with the ventricle; the mitral or bicuspid valve between the left atrium and left ventricle; and the aortic valve between the left ventricle and aorta. Mitral valve incompetence and aortic valvular disease result in the left ventricle having more blood within it and therefore having to work harder to pump blood around the body.

Another condition which makes the left ventricle work harder is **hypertension.** As the left ventricle has to contract with more force to pump the blood around the body it is more liable to fatigue. So a patient who suffers from hypertension overworks the left ventricle and therefore is more liable to left ventricular failure.

Signs and Symptoms

With these changes from normal physiology, the patient with left ventricular failure presents with:

A **low blood pressure** (hypotension) due to the failure of the left ventricle to pump the blood with any force.

A **rapid pulse** (tachycardia) due to the fact that the heart is beating faster to compensate for the low cardiac output and low blood pressure.

An **irregular heart beat** if the conducting mechanism has been disturbed by the ventricular heart muscle being damaged by lack of oxygen.

An **altered respiratory function** due to the extra fluid in the pulmonary circulation (produced by the back pressure of blood from the left side of the heart) causing pulmonary oedema. This oedema makes the patient's respirations sound moist and bubbly and a very watery sputum is produced. Due to the distress of breathing, the patient may be extremely anxious, pale, restless and in an exhausted state.

The patient will also **perspire** due to the effect of the sympathetic nervous system responding to the body's stress situation. The patient's general condition can be described as shocked due to the inadequate circulation caused by the low blood pressure.

The patient may have had some warning of left ventricular failure with a gradual build up of symptoms of breathlessness and increasing tiredness. However, in an acute attack of left ventricular failure the condition suddenly increases in severity and the patient requires immediate treatment.

Treatment

Acute left ventricular failure or cardiac asthma is treated with consideration for: breathing, circulation, oedema, pulmonary congestion, and anxiety and distress.

Breathing

To maintain the patient's breathing:
1   Ensure that the airway is clear.
2   Position the patient in a comfortable position to breathe easily, e.g., semirecumbent. Remember that although there may be breathing problems, you may not be able to sit the patient up because he or she may be hypotensive and an adequate circulation to the brain needs to be maintained.
3   Administer oxygen via a mask. Note whether the patient is cyanosed. The patient may be cyanosed due to the inadequate gaseous exchange in the lungs because of the pulmonary oedema.
4   Prepare drugs for administration to relieve the respiratory congestion, e.g., aminophylline.

Circulation

To observe and improve the patient's circulation:
1 Monitor the heart action by recording the pulse and blood pressure.
2 Monitor the patient's heart action by continuous ECG recordings.
3 Improve the heart circulation by administering drugs which will slow, steady and strengthen the heart action, e.g., digoxin.

Oedema

Oedema is controlled by the administration of diuretics, e.g., frusemide. It is essential to monitor the patient's urinary output in response to the diuretic therapy. This is to ensure the patient's kidneys are functioning adequately and are responding to the treatment. Hypotension with left ventricular failure will result in a decreased blood supply to the kidneys therefore their function may be inadequate.

Pulmonary Congestion

To relieve pulmonary congestion:
1 The patient may wish to sit with his or her legs dependent thereby limiting the amount of blood which circulates back to the right side of the heart.
2 Diuretic therapy used to control the oedema will relieve the pulmonary congestion.
3 The doctor may order that tourniquets are put on the limbs in order to reduce the venous return to the right side of the heart, thereby lessening the amount of blood entering the pulmonary circulation and reducing the pulmonary congestion (oedema). These tourniquets are applied on 3 limbs for a period of 15 minutes. One tourniquet is then released and applied to the fourth limb. This permits some circulation to the heart from the limbs and, by alternating the tourniquets around the limbs, allows circulation to the limbs.

Anxiety and Distress

It is necessary to try to relieve the patient's anxiety and distress. Reassurance and explanations aid the patient in these

situations, and is particularly important.
Anxiety is best relieved by a controlled drug such as morphine or diamorphine given intravenously, the dose being 10 - 15 mg. Remember that morphine has a side effect of causing respiratory depression.

Summary of Drugs

Drugs used in left ventricular failure may be made available by the nurse to be administered on the doctor's perscription. These include:
  Aminophylline — relieves respiratory congestion
  Digoxin — slows, steadies and strengthens heart action
  Frusemide — diuretic
  Morphine or diamorphine — relieves pain and anxiety

CONGESTIVE CARDIAC FAILURE

Congestive cardiac failure is not an acute condition but can be aggravated by acute left ventricular failure. It is the commonest chronic heart disease and is caused by the right side of the heart failing to function adequately.

Causes

Causes of congestive cardiac failure can be due to congenital heart conditions or any disease which puts extra stress on the right side of the heart. The diseases could be:
  Chronic pulmonary diseases
  Those that cause left ventricular failure (see p. 124).
Other conditions leading to congestive cardiac failure could be due to *thyrotoxicosis*. This is when the body's metabolism and activity are accelerated so that the heart is forced to work harder, and can therefore become more stressed.
Congestive cardiac failure manifests itself in a different way from left ventricular failure mainly because the pressure and accummulation of blood is in the right side of the heart. Blood is received into the right atrium from the superior and inferior vena cava (see Figure 36). From the atrium it passes via the

tricuspid valve to the right ventricle from which it is pumped via the pulmonary veins to the lungs. If the lungs are congested then the blood will accumulate in the pulmonary circulation, causing an alteration in capillary fluid exchange resulting in pulmonary oedema within the pulmonary circulation and in the right ventricle of the heart. This means that the right ventricle becomes distended.

If the right ventricle is not contracting adequately due to failure then again the ventricle becomes enlarged. The blood is unable to reach the lungs so that the oxygen levels are reduced and the patient becomes cyanosed. The accumulated blood causes back pressure and blood also collects in the right atrium and back into the venous circulation. As the pressure within the superior vena cava increases the jugular veins in the neck become distended (Figure 37). The pressure within the inferior vena cava results in the alteration of osmotic pressure in the venous capillaries and fluid remains in the tissues. The patient will then develop dependent oedema around the feet and buttocks.

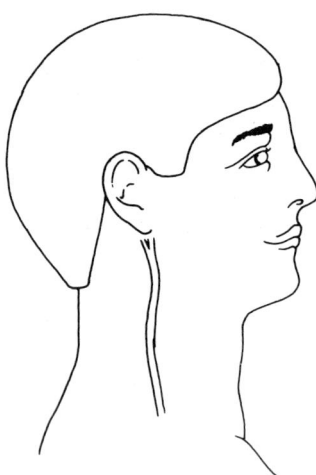

Figure 37 Position of the jugular vein. This vein becomes distended in congestive cardiac failure.

Signs and Symptoms

The patient may present in accident and emergency with symptoms due to respiratory distress or progressive heart failure.

These symptoms include:
 Tiredness
 Weakness
 Loss of appetite due to general body effects

Other effects due to the congestion include:
 Distended jugular veins
 Dependent oedema
 Enlarged liver
 Ascites
 Pleural effusion
 Diminished urinary output

The patient will also be cyanosed due to the poor circulation.

Treatment

The treatment is aimed at maintaining an adequate circulation with sufficient oxygen levels.

To maintain an adequate circulation:
1 Reduce fluid overload — diuretics.
2 Maintain heart function — digoxin.

To provide sufficient oxygen:
1 Sit patient upright with legs lowered to reduce venous return. It also helps to reduce oxygen consumption by resting the patient.
2 Give oxygen via a Ventimask at the correct concentration. This ensures that the patient is receiving adequate oxygen without a disturbance in the oxygen : carbon dioxide ratio within the patient's body.

Patients with the conditions discussed in this chapter are generally admitted into hospital for treatment.

REVISION OBJECTIVES

1 Describe and illustrate the normal structure and function of the heart.
2 Describe the normal structure of an artery and list the disorders that occur within the artery.
3 Discuss the condition of angina and myocardial infarction detailing signs, symptoms and treatment.
4 Describe the normal heart action and identify 5 abnormalities of heart action as shown on an electrocardiogram.

5   Outline the use of drugs and electrical defibrillation in heart disorders.
6   Describe the effects of left ventricular failure related to the signs and symptoms, discussing the nursing care and medical treatment.
7   Describe the condition of congestive cardiac failure; identify the effects and relate them to patient care and treatment.

6
Acute Respiratory Conditions

THE RESPIRATORY CENTRE

The respiratory centre which is located in the medulla oblongata in the brain stem controls the respiratory system. The respiratory system (Figure 38) is a tract extending from the

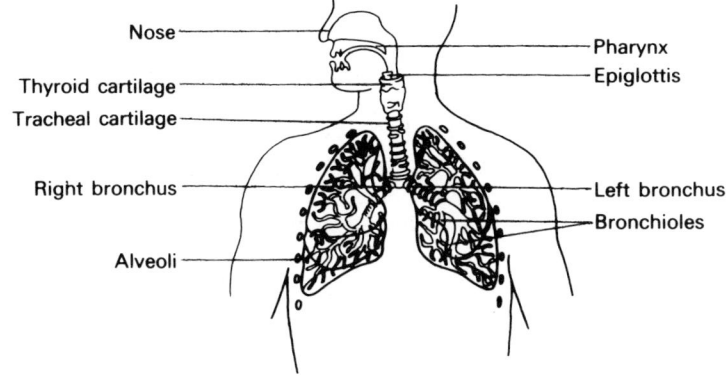

Figure 38 The respiratory system.

nostrils to the alveoli in the lungs. It is designed to clean and warm the air and allow the air to pass to the alveoli where gaseous exchange takes place.

The respiratory centre adjusts respiratory activity mainly through the influence of the carbon dioxide levels in the blood. As the carbon dioxide level increases so does the respiratory rate. Oxygen shortage on the other hand can also indirectly stimulate the respiratory centre. Oxygen levels are approximately 4 kPa - 8 kPa before this stimulus functions.

Causes of Alteration

Causes of alteration in the respiratory centre's function:

Depression of respirations due to an overdose of drugs which depress the respiratory centre, e.g., anaesthetics or control drugs such as morphine.

Damage directly or indirectly to the respiratory centre in the medulla oblongata:

Head injury — Actual damage to the medulla oblongata or pressure caused by cerebral swelling or haemorrhage.

Cerebral vascular accidents may also directly or indirectly disturb the respiratory centre, due to damage or swelling.

Changes in Respiratory Function

Changes in respiratory function may be a result of alteration of the respiratory centre.

Hypoventilation

Hypoventilation is diminished breathing which results in inadequate total alveolar ventilation.

Treatment. Treatment involves the use of drugs to stimulate the respiratory centre, e.g., narcan, nikethamide.

Cheyne-Stokes Respiration

Cheyne-Stokes respiration is an alteration in the rate and depth of respiration alternating from noisy and rapid respirations to quiet, deep, slow respirations. It is thought that this disturbance is due to an inability of the respiratory centre to act on the levels of carbon dioxide in the blood. Quiet, deep, slow respirations allow carbon dioxide levels to rise in the blood. When these levels reach a certain height the respiratory centre is stimulated and noisy, rapid respirations result.

Treatment. Treatment involves dealing with the cause if possible. Raised intracranial pressure disrupting the function of the medulla oblongata may possibly be relieved by drugs or surgery (see Chapter 8). Cheyne-Stokes respiration is usually a poor sign and the only treatment if necessary will be by mechanical ventilation.

Hyperventilation

Hyperventilation is an increase in the rate of respiration. The blood carbon dioxide levels are being decreased because the rapid respiration is expelling carbon dioxide from the body. The condition of hyperventilation if untreated can lead to a disturbance in the electrolyte balance. The patient may complain of dizziness and sensations of tingling or numbness around the mouth and in the hands. The patient may even demonstrate carpopedal spasm.

Treatment. The treatment of hyperventilation is to replace the carbon dioxide. This can be done by making the patient breath in his or her own carbon dioxide. Place a paper bag over the patient's nose and mouth and ask the patient to breath in and out of the bag. Remember the condition is usually precipitated by an emotional upset so if the patient can be calmed and reassured the actual hyperventilation will decrease.

The Mechanism of Respiration

Within the larger arteries of the thoracic cavity, the carotid and aorta, there are special cells that are sensitive to the amount of carbon dioxide in the blood (normal amount of CO_2 is 5.3 kPa).

When blood levels of CO_2 rise, impulses are passed from these specialized cells via cranial nerves to the respiratory centre. The nerves responsible for the conduction of the impulses are two of the cranial nerves: the ninth pair — glossopharyngeal nerves and the tenth pair — the vagus nerves.

Once the message of an increasing CO_2 level has reached the respiratory centre the impulse is conveyed by two nerves back to the thoracic cavity. The phrenic nerve goes to the diaphragm and the intercostal nerves go to the intercostal muscles. These impulses cause the muscles to contract and allow inspiration to occur.

Inspiration

Inspiration is the first stage of respiration.

The phrenic nerve stimulates the diaphragm to contract so it flattens. The intercostal nerves stimulate the intercostal muscle to contract which moves the rib cage up and out. The movement of these muscles stretches the lungs with them and decreases the pressure within the thoracic cavity. This allows air from the atmosphere to rush into the lungs to equalize the pressure. When air has entered the lungs the process of inspiration is complete (Figure 39a).

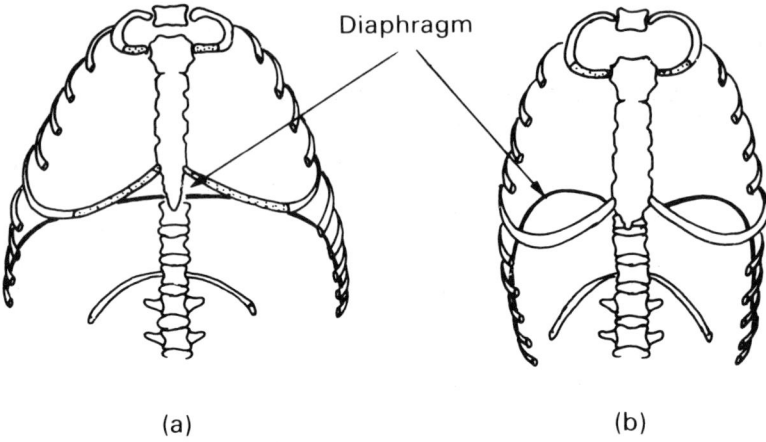

(a)   (b)

Figure 39 The respiratory mechanism: inspiration (a); expiration (b).

Expiration

Expiration consists of a relaxation of the muscles. It may be influenced by the reflex mechanism. Once the lungs have reached a certain capacity of air then a message is sent via the vagus nerves back to the respiratory centre to initiate relaxation of the muscles.

In expiration the intercostal muscles relax and return the ribs to their original position and the diaphragm relaxes and comes up to its normal dome shape (Figure 39b). This results in a decrease in the size of the thoracic cavity and forces the air out, which is expiration.

Voluntary Control of Respiration

The cerebral cortex is the area of the brain which is responsible for the control of voluntary movement of the chest (see Chapter 8) so that a person can consciously control the rate and depth of respiration. Other muscles are involved in respiration, i.e., when taking a deep breath or when there is difficulty in breathing.

These muscles are skeletal muscles known as the accessory muscles of respiration.

On inspiration the sternomastoid and the pectoralis muscles contract to raise the upper ribs and so enlarge the thoracic cavity.

On expiration the abdominal muscles contract to move the diaphragm back to its original dome shape.

Table 4 The difference between inspired and expired air.

Content	Inspired (%)	Expired (%)
Oxygen	20	16
Carbon Dioxide	0.04	4
Nitrogen	79.96	80

Inspired air contains 0.5% water vapour
Expired air contains 6.2% water vapour

Other factors which may influence the control of respiration include variations in temperature, presence of pain, or emotional situations.

The **temperature** control of the body is in the hypothalamus, this may stimulate the respiratory centre.

Pain can act as a stimulant to breathing. When a child is born it might initially be smartly smacked between the shoulder blades to produce respiration. Chest or upper abdominal pain may specially influence the rate and depth of respirations, tending to make them shallow and rapid. The increase in respiration is due largely to the sympathetic nervous system stimulation.

Emotional situations can be upsetting, often lead to over-breathing (hyperventilation).

Alteration in the Mechanism

Alterations in the mechanism of respiration are produced by conditions which alter the functioning of the nerves and thoracic cavity, e.g., trauma, rib fractures, nerve damage, stab wounds. Altered nerve function can be due to disease, e.g., polio, myasthenia gravis.

Treatment. The treatment in the case of injury to the chest wall, is to support the chest by firm bandages. Rib fractures are usually allowed to heal on their own unless they are causing damage to internal structures (see Chapter 4 on thoracic injuries).

If the mechanics of respiration are sufficiently damaged or diseased then artificial means of ventilation must be instituted immediately.

Obstruction to the airway is a cause of hypoventilation and can occur at any point in the respiratory tract. Upper airway obstructions have been discussed (see Chapter 3).

LOWER AIRWAY OBSTRUCTION

Obstruction of the lower parts of the airway are due to disease:
Asthma
Bronchitis

Asthma

Asthma is a fairly common condition seen in the accident and emergency department. In normal physiology, on inspiration atmospheric air rushes into the respiratory tract and on expiration the air is forced out. However, with asthma:
- The smooth involuntary muscle of the bronchi of the lungs has contracted causing muscle spasm.
- The inflammatory reaction can result in mucosal swelling, causing further constriction of the bronchioles.
- Excess secretions obstruct and narrow the bronchi.
- Air is trapped within the alveoli as it is unable to be expired sufficiently.

Causes of Asthma

The causes of asthma are:
- Often unknown — idiopathic
- Emotional
- Environmental — due to allergic reactions to allergens such as dust mites, pollen, fur etc.
- Chest infection

Signs and Symptoms

A patient with asthma will present with dyspnoea, wheezing, coughing with sputum, perspiring, nausea and possible cyanosis. A patient has **dyspnoea** because of difficulty in expiring air due to the narrowing of the lumen of the bronchi.

The characteristic **wheeze** is the sound made as air is forced through the bronchi when the patient exhales. In an asthmatic patient the wheeze is related to expiration.

Coughing and **sputum** are due to the inflammatory response occurring in the bronchi and the patient produces sticky sputum. Ensure that the patient has a sputum pot and tissues. Keep a specimen of sputum for bacterial examination.

Perspiration and **nausea** will be experienced by any patient who is having difficulty in breathing. The patient may be extremely anxious and tense.

Cyanosis may result from severe or prolonged disturbance in oxygen exchange.

Treatment

Asthma **must** be recognized and the patient treated immediately.

1. Sit the patient upright and loosen tight clothing around the neck, chest and waist. The patient will be using the accessory muscles and abdominal muscles to aid respiration.
2. Allow the patient a feeling of space; open the door or the window in warm weather to allow the patient air. The patient's anxiety will be increased if he or she feels claustrophobic.
3. Assess the patient. Observe the blood pressure, pulse, respirations and temperature. It is advisable to take an axilla temperature or in children a rectal temperature. In the acute stage the patient will be too distressed to have a thermometer in his or her mouth because of having to breathe through the mouth.
4. Summon the doctor.
5. Reassurance may aid in calming the patient. Remember, one of the causes of asthma is emotional. However, drugs will be required to relax the bronchial muscle.
6. Oxygen may be given to the patient. This is not always essential in the acute attack as hypoxia is not usually severe. However, oxygen may psychologically help the patient.

Administration of Oxygen. Oxygen is generally administered by nasal spectacles, in this case at the rate of 2 - 4 litres per minute, as the patient who has dyspnoea often cannot tolerate an oxygen mask over the face. Oxygen, if administered, must be humidified to prevent drying of respiratory tract mucosa.

Alternatively, intermittent positive pressure breathing (IPPB) can be used to administer oxygen. If the patient can manage to use this apparatus it enables a volume of air to be forcefully directed into the lungs. It also allows drugs to be administered directly into the respiratory tract, e.g., salbutamol (Ventolin) which relax bronchial muscle. The IPPB also helps to loosen secretions in the bronchi and allows them to be expectorated thereby clearing the respiratory tract.

Drug Therapy

Aminophylline 250 mg is given intravenously initially. (This may be given by oral or rectal administration if the patient is not severely distressed). It is an antispasmodic drug and should relax the bronchospasm within 20 minutes. An important side effect is cardiac arrhythmias. For this reason the patient's pulse must be monitored at 15-minute intervals.

Adrenaline 1:1000 is an antispasmodic drug producing bronchodilatation, but has side effects.

One of these two drugs is generally used to treat an acute asthmatic attack and should be effective within 20 minutes. This means that the doctor will re-examine the patient within 20 minutes. If the patient has not sufficiently improved then a repeat dose of the drug will be given. These drugs are generally only repeated twice.

Steroids. Another group of drugs which may be used are steroids. Steroids are anti-inflammatory drugs and are therefore useful in suppressing the inflammatory response within the lungs. However, they are not administered unless necessary due to the side effects they can produce. Steroids will be administered to the acute asthmatic patient who is on steroid therapy continuously.

In times of stress to the body in normal health the adrenal glands function and produce the glucocorticoids whenever they are needed. For the patient on steroid therapy the action of the adrenal glands has been suppressed so that they are unable to produce extra steroids in times of stress. Therefore, increased drug doses are required. That is why it is so important that the doctor is aware that a patient is on steroid therapy. Lack of corticoids produces hypotension and hypoglycaemia.

For other patients' steroid therapy will be commenced when they are no longer responding to the aminophylline or adrenaline. Corticoid can be used in an acute attack.

Hydrocortisone acetate 100 mg intravenously every 4 hours will bring the attack under control. It must be slowly decreased over several days, giving prednisolone 100 - 30 mg daily. Do **not** allow the patient to use his or her own prescribed drugs or inhalers during the acute treatment as this will disturb the action of the drugs the doctor is giving.

Intravenous Therapy

Therapy involving the use of an intravenous infusion may be commenced for drug administration and also to maintain the fluid balance.

Patients may become dehydrated due to:
   An inability to drink due to dyspnoea
   Nausea and vomiting
   Excess secretion of water in respiration. The normal amount of water excreted via the respiratory tract is 500 ml in 24 hours.

Following treatment the patient may be admitted to hospital or discharged home. Long term treatment involves treating the underlying cause, e.g., infection or allergy.

Acute asthma attacks which are not controlled by drugs within 24 hours progress to the condition of status asthmaticus. The patient will have been admitted to hospital in this case and may require mechanical ventilation to maintain blood gases within normal limits and prevent the patient becoming extremely exhausted.

Bronchitis

Bronchitis is an inflammatory reaction within the bronchi of the lungs. Bronchitis may occur suddenly (acute) or be progressive (chronic). The accident and emergency department tends to see the acute attack of bronchitis because the patients are sufficiently distressed to require immediate treatment. Patients with chronic bronchitis can live a modified normal life within the limits of their breathlessness. However, patients with chronic bronchitis may present in the department due to a sudden deterioration in their condition which has produced an acute attack on top of a chronic condition.

Causes

The causes of bronchitis are:
 Generally an upper respiratory tract infection often due to a virus, e.g., cold.
 Smoke atmospheres
 Cold, damp conditions

Physiology of Bronchitis

Bronchitis is an inflammatory response of the lining of the bronchi. As in all inflammatory reactions there is local vasodilatation and increased fluid and leucocytes in the tissues. In the bronchi this produces sputum.

Signs and Symptoms

A patient with bronchitis will present with the following signs and symptoms:
 Breathlessness
 Dyspnoea
 Elevated temperature
 A feeling of tightness and soreness within the chest. This is due to the irritation of nerve endings by the inflammatory reaction.
 Cough — further aggravating the soreness of the chest.
 Sputum — which may be thick and tenacious and which may also contain bacteria. The patient may have a haemoptysis or sputum may be tinged with blood. The inflammatory process has allowed erythrocytes to filter from the blood capillaries into the bronchi from where they are expectorated.
 Cyanosis — Due to the blockage within the bronchi air is unable to reach the alveoli for adequate oxygen exchange.

Treatment

Treatment of acute bronchitis:
1 Sit the patient upright and loosen tight clothing around neck, chest and waist.
2 Observe the patient. Record the blood pressure, pulse, respirations and temperature.
3 Observe for cyanosis. Oxygen may be administered but with extreme caution. Patients with chronic bronchitis have adapted to a high level of carbon dioxide in their blood, and this high level is their respiratory stimulant. By administering oxygen the carbon dioxide level in the blood may be reduced sufficiently to cause respiratory depression.
Administer oxygen via a Ventimask if necessary at a rate of 24 %.
4 Provide the patient with a sputum carton and tissues. Obtain a specimen of sputum for laboratory investigation.
5 The bronchospasm will be relieved by aminophylline 250 mg intravenously.

Another disease causing lower airway obstruction is pulmonary oedema (see Chapter 5).

REVISION OBJECTIVES

1 Illustrate the respiratory system.
2 Describe the normal control of the respiratory system and identify alterations in the function of the respiratory centre.
3 Describe the mechanism of respiration.
4 Relate the signs and symptoms of asthma to the physiological changes and describe the methods of patient care and treatment of the acute attack.
5 Describe the condition of bronchitis, relate the signs and symptoms to the treatment.

7
Disturbances in Skin Function and Body Surface Trauma

THE SKIN

The skin is the outer covering to the body and as such it is liable to a diversity of injuries from various causes (see also Chapter 4).

Structure

The skin is composed of two layers: the epidermis — outer layer and the dermis — inner layer (Figure 40).

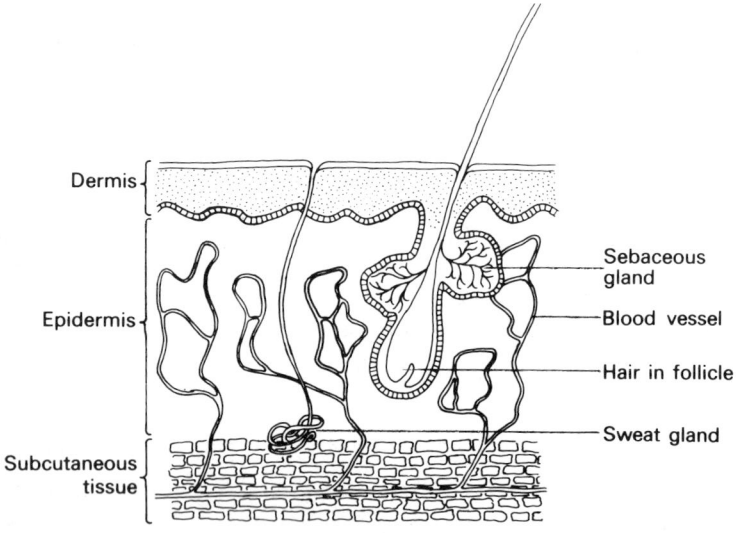

Figure 40 The structure of the skin.

Epidermis

The *epidermis* consists of several layers of cells which vary in appearance and thickness. These cells form the tissue of the skin known as squamous epithelium. The cells contain:

Keratin — a substance which hardens the cells and protects the deeper layers.
Melanin — a colour pigment.
Deeper cells are capable of dividing rapidly so that they move up and replace the flatter more worn cells at the surface which are shed by any form of friction on the skin.
The epidermis contains no blood vessels or nerves.

Dermis

The dermis consists of fibrous tissue and elastic fibres which enable the skin to move and stretch especially around joints in the body. The dermis contains:
Blood vessels.
Lymphatic vessels.
Glands. These glands include:
Sweat glands which secrete water and salts to maintain the water and electrolyte balance.
Sebaceous glands which secrete an oily substance (sebum).
The sebum is discharged into the hair follicle (see Figure 40) and keeps the hair shiny and soft. Sebum also aids in waterproofing the skin and protecting the skin against bacteria.
Hair follicles. A hair follicle allows the hair to grow within it and small muscles attached to the hair follicle allow the hair to stand on end.
Nerve endings. Nerve endings allow the skin to perform its function as a sense organ. The nerves respond to sensations of pain, heat, cold, pressure, and fine touch. These sensations are the beginning of a reflex action (see Chapter 8).
Under the skin is the subcutaneous tissue which contains fat cells and connects with the underlying muscles.

Abrasions and Burns. The structure of the skin must be considered in the treatment of minor injuries such as abrasions or in the case of burns.
1 If the patient bleeds from the abrasion then the damage to the skin has gone deeper than the epidermis.
2 If the damage to the tissue involves the epidermis and the superficial layer of the dermis, such as in the case of a superficial burn, then the patient will feel pain recorded by the nerve endings in the dermis.

3   If a patient with skin damage, such as a burn, does not feel pain then the tissue damage is deeper and more severe because the nerves in the dermis have been completely destroyed.

FUNCTIONS

The skin functions as:
Protection. Protection against:
   Wear and tear
   Water
   Bateria
   Ultraviolet rays of the sun. This function is maintained by the melanin in the skin which also gives skin its colour. This deepens to form a suntan during exposure.
A **sensory organ.**
An **excretory organ.** As an excretory organ, the sweat glands aid in the removal of waste material.
Vitamin D formation. Vitamin D is formed from a substance in the sebum with the aid of ultraviolet rays on the skin. Lack of vitamin D causes rickets.
A **heat regulator.** Heat regulation is controlled by the hypothalamus in the brain. The skin aids in cooling the body in warm weather in two ways:
1   The blood vessels to the skin dilate and more blood is circulated to the skin surface.
2   The increase of blood to the skin enables the sweat glands to excrete more water and salt.

Disturbances in Skin Function

Heat Exhaustion

In especially hot climates the perspiration produced by the sweat glands can result in a disturbance of water and electrolyte balance in the body, known as *heat exhaustion.*

Signs and Symptoms. In heat exhaustion the patient complains of a headache, dizziness, tiredness, nausea and possibly cramp pains. The patient is generally perspiring and will appear pale and clammy. The patient may present in a condition of shock, because the peripheral blood vessels are dilated and blood is circulating in the peripheral blood vessels and the amount reaching the brain and heart is diminished. The patient will present with hypotension and tachycardia.

Treatment. Treatment for heat exhaustion:
1   Treat the shock by placing the patient in a recumbent position with legs elevated.
2   Remove the cause. Move the patient to a cool place. Keep the patient cool.
3   Replace the lost fluid. This should be done by using intravenous solutions of normal saline given at a rate of about 200 ml an hour.

Do **not** give oral fluids especially if the patient is nauseated, as this will only produce vomiting and further fluid loss from the body.

Body Temperature

The normal body temperature is 37.4°C (98.4°F). This is maintained by 2 actions.
1   The hypothalamus stimulates the nervous system to produce muscular action. This action creates shivering. The hair on the skin surface also stands on end during shivering which allows warm air to be trapped near to the skin surface. For muscles to move they require oxygen and glucose from the blood. Once the oxygen and glucose has been used carbon dioxide and heat are produced. Carbon dioxide is excreted from the body via the lungs and the heat produced raises the body temperature.
2   The blood vessels in the skin constrict, so blood circulates in the larger vessels and maintains the temperature of blood passing through the heart to the brain. Remember that blood coming to the peripheral skin blood vessels cools the body temperature.

Temperature within the body varies. The core of the body, the centre which contains the vital organs, is warmer; the peripheral area of the body is cooler. Because the core of the body contains the vital organs it is important that this temperature is:
1   Recorded accurately. The most accurate method of taking the core temperature is rectally.
2   Maintained within normal limits (35–37.4°C).

Temperature Disturbances

Heat Stroke

The patient who presents with a sudden rise in temperature to 41°C has *heat stroke*.

Signs and Symptoms. This patient will **not** perspire. The skin is hot, dry and flushed in appearance. The condition untreated will progress to seizures or unconsciousness. This disorder is a disturbance in the heat-regulating centre in the brain — the hypothalamus.

Treatment. The treatment of heat stroke requires the nurse to:
1 Maintain an airway.
2 Move the patient to a cool environment:
   Use a fan to cool the air.
   With tepid water, sponge the patient to lower the temperature.
3 Maintain the circulation by administering the lost fluid intravenously.
4 Record observations of blood pressure, pulse, respirations and temperature at half-hourly intervals.

In Britain, heat exhaustion or heat stroke is not often caused by the excessive temperature of the climate but by conditions of work. The people most susceptible to this, e.g., boiler workers or firemen, work in hot, humid environments.

The skin also aids in the reaction of the body to the cold.

Hypothermia

If the body temperature is below 35°C then the patient has *hypothermia*. The heat-regulating centre is no longer functioning satisfactorily.

Causes. Causes of hypothermia can be:
   Exposure
   Immobility — muscle activity creates heat
   Disease which slows the body metabolism — *myxoedema*

Signs and Symptoms. The signs and symptoms with which to recognize hypothermia include:
   Cold to touch
   Rectal temperature below 35°C

Sluggish in movement
Drowsiness, confusion or alteration in conscious level
Signs of oxygen depletion

Due to the lowered body temperature the basal metabolic action of the body is decreased. Cells require less oxygen as they slow down. However, as the temperature becomes lower (34°C) the vital control centres are unable to function efficiently. The alterations include:
Slow respiration
Irregular heart action
 such as atrial fibrillation.

The effect of this heart irregularity is to present a patient in the condition of shock.

Cardiac arrest may occur when the core temperature is below 31°C.

Treatment. The overall treatment is to warm the patient gradually.

1 Place the patient in a warm room.
2 Remove any wet or cold clothing. It is important to wash the patient's skin and dry it thoroughly if the skin is wet from water or incontinence.
3 Cover the patient with warm blankets. The patient may be completely wrapped in a hypothermia blanket. This blanket is made of foil and can be wrapped immediately around the patient. Blankets can then be placed over the patient.
4 If the patient is conscious and has a swallowing reflex give a **warm**, not hot drink.
5 The patient should not be rewarmed at more than 0.5°C an hour. Rapid rewarming can further disturb the temperature control centre.
6 Regular observation of blood pressure, pulse, respirations and temperature, taken rectally at hourly intervals. Treatment may be required due to cardiac involvement. To observe the heart's changes the patient may be connected to a heart monitor. Treatment will depend on the arrhythmia (see Chapter 5).
7 Administer antibiotics. Following hypothermia patients are susceptible to infections especially chest infections. Treatment is usually commenced prophylactically initially with ampicillin.

Ensure that:
1 The patient is **not** given a hot water bottle.
2 The patient is **not** placed touching a radiator. Remember due to the general slowing of the body metabolism the reactions of the body to sensations are also diminished. These patients can suffer from burns due to heat being applied directly to them.
3 The patient is **not** given hot drinks. Hot drinks will cause dilation of the blood vessels of the gastrointestinal tract, this will remove blood from the vital organs and result in further cooling.
4 The patient is **not** given alcohol. Alcohol dilates the peripheral blood vessels and so removes blood from the core of the body. As blood circulates through the peripheral blood vessels it is cooled. Alcohol will aggravate the condition of hypothermia.

BODY SURFACE TRAUMA

Burns

A burn is the exposure of the body to heat which is sufficient to cause damage to the skin and underlying tissues. It is caused by excessive heat or low heat for long periods.

Causes

Burns can be caused by:
  Chemicals
  Friction
  Heat
  Dry — the flame of a fire
  Moist — from hot liquid scalds
  Electrical — as the electrical current travels through the patient it results in burns at the point of contact, e.g., hands, and at the point of exit when the current stops, e.g., soles of feet. These patients often have 2 separate areas of burns
The severity of the burn and its effects on the patient are variable.

Table 5 Wallace's rule of nine.

Area of body	%
Head	9
1 Arm	9
1 Leg	
Back	9
Front	9
Chest	9
Back	9
Abdomen	9
Buttocks	9
Perineum	1

Estimation

Estimation of the burnt area depends on the area burnt and the depth of the burn. The burnt area is estimated in several ways:

With **Wallace's rule of nine**, the body is divided into areas of approximately 9 % (Table 5).

With **rule of hand**, the patient's hand (fingers closed and palm) is estimated as 1 % of the total skin surface.

Special **charts** have been designed for greater accuracy, e.g., Lund and Browder.

Depth

The depth of skin loss to the area marked 'partial skin loss' (Figure 41) can be determined by the patient's response to a pin prick. Sensitivity to the pin prick will indicate that the nerves of the dermis are still intact so the patient has only *partial skin loss*. No response to the pin prick means that the nerves of the dermis are no longer intact and the patient has *whole skin loss*. A burnt area can often be a mixture of partial and whole skin loss. Minor burns are discussed in chapter 4.

Severe burns require highly specialized treatment and should, when possible, be transferred to the nearest burns unit, where facilities and staff are available. This means that severe burns are not often seen in the accident and emergency departments of hospitals in Britain.

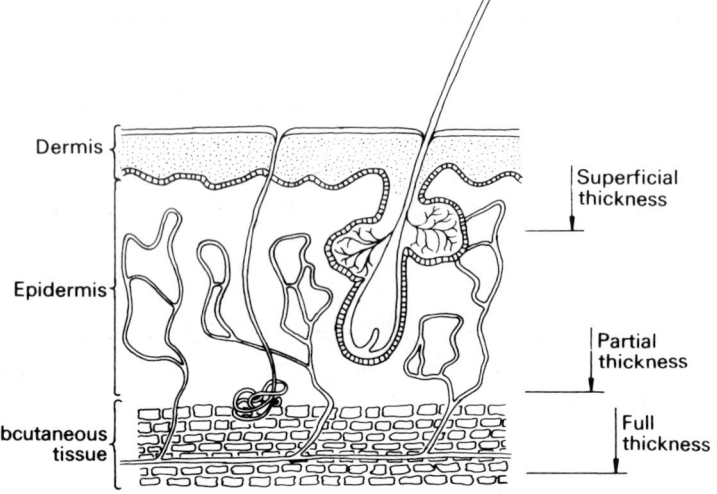

Figure 41 The structure of the skin showing the depth of injury related to burns.

Treatment

Treatment follows priorities:
Before commencing treatment, ensure that the patient is breathing and has a pulse.
Maintain the airway especially in cases of burns around the throat area. Local oedema may cause obstruction. Burns to the upper airway may necessitate a tracheostomy to maintain ventilation.
Maintain breathing as smoke can affect the lungs although not always directly. The patient may complain of dyspnoea and chest pain. Alteration in the respiratory function may require intubation and mechanical ventilation. Be aware that the irritant reaction to the smoke or burn may result in oedema of the respiratory tract and respiratory distress several hours after the initial incident. Fifteen minute observations of respirations are important. The patient with suspected smoke inhalation will be admitted for observation for a 24 to 48 hour period.

Shock. The severely burned patient will develop hypovolaemic shock due to the loss of plasma from the burned areas of the skin. The patient often complains of thirst but **do not** give anything by mouth without consulting the doctor. The patient may complain of nausea and vomiting. Shock **must** be recognized and treated. To recognize shock take blood pressure and pulse recordings. These may be recorded on the arm or leg, depending on the area burnt. Estimation of the burned area will indicate the severity of the patient's condition. This estimation is conducted using special charts, haematocrit and clinical judgement.

A shock case is defined as:
  A child with 10 % or more of the total skin surface destroyed.
  An adult with 15 % or more of the total skin surface destroyed.

Treatment:
  Blood samples taken by doctor
  Replacing fluid loss with intravenous infusion of plasma or Human Plasma Protein Fraction (HPPF).

Electrolyte Changes. Electrolyte changes must be corrected or certain conditions may result:
  Hypokalaemia — Low potassium level. The potassium may be lost due to vomiting.
  Hypocalcaemia — Deficiency of blood calcium. This results in the condition of tetany. Calcium gluconate will be administered intravenously.

Prevention of Infection

A burns unit has a special sterile room to help prevent infection. Infection is a serious complication of burns. The area for carrying out dressing must be carefully considered. The aseptic cleaning and dressing of the burn must be decided by the doctor. In some instances the burn may be left exposed and the patient started on antibiotic therapy. Tetanus toxoid and Humotet may be given.

If the patient has a partial skin loss then the burn is extremely painful. Analgesia, generally a controlled drug, will be ordered by the doctor.

Prevention of Deformity

To prevent deformity through the development of contractions positioning of the burnt area is important. When positioning any joints they must be in a position of extension.

Other Injuries. The patient may have other injuries apart from the burn, e.g., the patient may have been involved in a road traffic accident when the car ignited. Assess the priorities and treat the patient accordingly.

Catheterization. The patient may require catheterization especially if burns are around the perineum. A strict aseptic technique is required. Catheterization is also required to record an accurate urinary output. In all cases of shock blood is circulated primarily to the vital organs, the brain and heart. There is a decreased blood volume to the kidneys resulting in decreased kidney function. In severe cases of shock the patient may develop acute renal failure.

Stress. Bleeding of the gastrointestinal tract may result within a few hours of the burn. This is a rare condition believed to be due to the body's reaction to stress. The patient will require a blood transfusion.

When 20% of the body is involved, the patient may develop *hypochromic anaemia* at a later stage. Anaemia is a deficiency in the quality or quantity of erythrocytes. In this case the cells are small with insufficient haemoglobin formed. This may be due to initial damage to the erythrocytes or as a result of the body's reaction to stress.

Treatment of Specific Burns

Some specific burns, i.e., electrical or chemical need particular treatment:

Electrical burns may cause a cardiac arrest or ventricular fibrillation. **Resuscitate** immediately. Later problems may involve tissue necrosis or progressive thrombosis due to initial damage to blood vessels.

Chemicals are irritants and need to be removed as soon as possible. They may be washed off with water. If the chemical is an acid use weak vinegar. If the chemical is an alkaline use sodium bicarbonate.

Psychological Care

The psychological care of the patient must be considered. Burns are disfiguring although plastic surgery has made many advances in their care and eventual outcome. However, a patient with burns can still be very distressed.

Advice to the nurse:
1 Do not let your distress be obvious to a patient who is being observed by you.
2 Try to reassure the patient by explaining care. In some cases the patient will be unable to see due to damage to the eyes or oedema of the eyelids.
3 Ensure that the patient knows when you are present.
4 Relieve the pain. Administer analgesia when ordered.
5 Give all ordered treatment in a calm manner.
6 Listen to the patient. Assessing the situation of the incident is important. Knowing how the patient received the injury may indicate some of the psychological needs of the patient.
The circumstances which lead to the burns may result in additional psychological problems.

Road Traffic Accident. A road traffic accident may involve several people. The patient may have caused the accident or may be concerned about the other people in the car.

House Fire. With a house fire, the patient may be anxious about other family members. The fire may mean that the patient may be homeless.
When the patient's condition is satisfactory he or she should be allowed to see other family members. This can often be an emotional experience for all. Relatives must be warned about a patient's condition before being shown in. Whenever possible make sure that relatives are informed about the patient's progress while they are waiting in the department.
It is advisable when several members of the family are waiting to see the doctor to allow them to wait in the same cubicle. Only the patient who requires urgent treatment should be treated in a separate area. Waiting together helps to relieve anxiety.
The homeless patient will require social services.
The patient bereaved because of the fire will require psychological and spiritual help.

If children have lost their parents due to the fire they will require special care and may be detained in hospital until social services have made arrangments for their care.

Suicide Attempt. Some people set fire to themselves in a suicide attempt. Such a situation must be recognized as this patient will require both physical and psychological treatment. Once the physical condition has stabilized, the patient will be referred to a psychiatrist for further treatment.

REVISION OBJECTIVES

1   Describe and illustrate the structure and function of the skin.
2   Detail the signs and symptoms of heat exhaustion and heat stroke and the methods of patient care and treatment required.
3   Describe the effects of hypothermia and administer the required patient care.
4   List the causes of burns.
5   State ways to estimate the burnt area.
6   Describe the treatment of burns in order of priority.
7   Discuss the psychological effects of burns.

8
The Unconscious Patient

UNCONSCIOUSNESS

Unconsciousness can be likened to a deep abnormal sleep of unknown duration from which a patient cannot be roused no matter what stimulus is used. Unconsciousness cannot be measured directly only the levels of consciousness (see p.23).

The vital factor regarding unconsciousness from the nursing viewpoint is that the patient is without some or all reflex actions. The reflex actions are:
Swallowing
Coughing
Blinking
Pain
Continence

The most important reflex action is swallowing. The nurse **must** be alert to the fact that the patient's tongue may fall backwards, thereby obstructing the airway.

THE NERVOUS SYSTEM

The reticular formation situated in the brain stem is the area within the nervous system which is responsible for our conscious level. The nervous system works as a whole but can be divided into 3 main parts.
   Central nervous system which comprises the brain and the
      spinal cord.
   Peripheral nervous system which consists of the spinal nerves
      forming the reflex arc.
   Automonic nervous system which is divided into 2 parts:
      Sympathetic nervous system
      Parasympathetic nervous system
The nervous system is divided into these groups because of the

various functions it has to maintain. Although the groups have separate functions they are also related and even overlap in some functions.

Autonomic Nervous System

The autonomic nervous system is the system which keeps the body functioning on a 24-hour basis. It is responsible for the involuntary actions, the actions not consciously thought about, e.g., digestion and the peristaltic action of the bowel.

It is the **parasympathetic** system which is relied on for the normal day to day body functions.

The **sympathetic** nervous system works in contrast and, as stated in many books, is the system of flight, fright and fight and is the body's reaction in times of stress. Consider the things which happen to you when you are frightened, your

Mouth becomes dry and sticky
Heart beats quicker
Muscles become tense
Pupils enlarge

All these are effects of the sympathetic nervous system. Another effect which is more noticeable in animals, is the way in which the hair stands on end. So the sympathetic nervous system allows the body to make a quick reaction to a situation.

Peripheral Nervous System

The peripheral nervous system also allows a quick reaction by its reflex action (see chapter 9). Reflex actions are recorded as conscious actions by the central nervous system, so the nervous systems work together. The reticular formation in the central nervous system causes unconsciousness and as the central nervous system is disturbed any of its functions can be disturbed also, i.e., a loss of some or all of the reflex actions.

Central Nervous System

The central nervous system (Figure 42) consists of the brain and the spinal cord but with unconsciousness it is the functions of the brain that need to be considered. The brain is divided into 3 main parts:

Cerebrum which is the largest part.

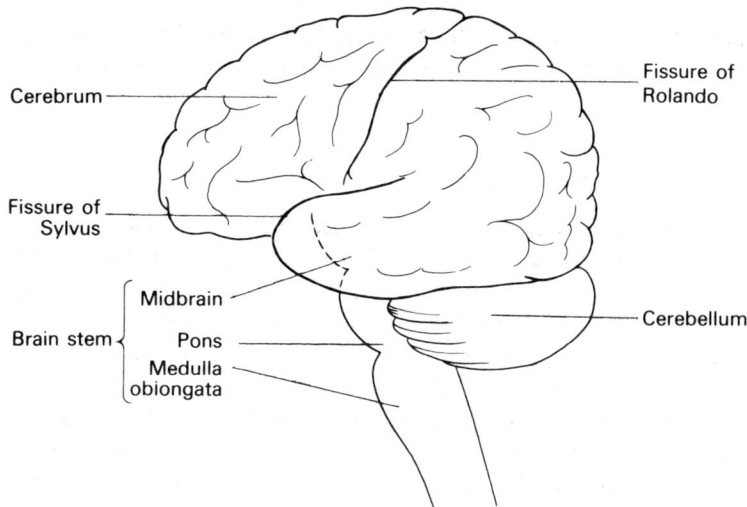

Figure 42 The central nervous system.

Cerebellum which is the smaller part and is beneath the cerebrum posteriorly.
Brain stem which consists of three areas:
Midbrain
Pons
Medulla oblongata

Damage to any part of the brain can disturb the functions of the medulla oblongata.

Functions of the Cerebrum

The cerebrum is divided into 4 separate areas (Figure 43), i.e., the parietal lobe, the frontal lobe, the temporal lobe and the occipital lobe.

Parietal lobe. The sensation of heat or cold, sharp or dull may be recorded in the **parietal lobe**. The sensation of pain may be registered here although it is thought a group of cells in the brain known as the **thalamus** register pain stimuli. The area which discharges impulses involving movement corresponds with the area of sensation in the parietal area and is found in the frontal lobe in the motor area. In order to alter a reflex action, the impulse must pass from the parietal area through the motor area and then down the spinal cord to the motor neurone of the reflex arc.

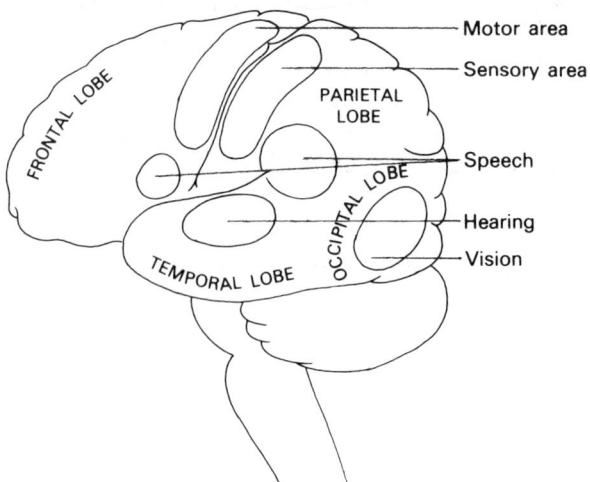

Figure 43 The central nervous system showing areas of function without the cerebrum.

Both the parietal and frontal lobe are responsible for speech. The parietal lobe is believed to control the interpretation of speech so that a person uses the correct words to express what is intended to be said.

The **frontal lobe** is responsible for the movement of speech, so that if a patient cannot form the words or speak clearly there may be a problem with the frontal lobe of the cerebrum.

The **temporal lobe** is responsible for the sensation of hearing and balance and also emotions, thoughts, mood and possibly musical appreciation.

The **occipital lobe** is responsible for sight.

Other Areas within the Cerebrum. Within the cerebrum are groups of nerve cells which have highly specialized functions. Part of their functions are to act as relay stations. As relay stations they have 2 main actions:

To decide whether a message (stimulus) is important enough to be passed on.

To conduct the message (stimulus) to the correct part of the brain for action to occur.

Some of these cells also have important individual functions:

The **basal ganglia** cells influence the tone of skeletal muscle.

The **thalamus** receives all sensory impulses, those messages from the peripheral nerves concerned with sensations of pain, temperature, pressure and touch and relays the messages to the cerebral cortex.

The **hypothalamus** is a small group of cells situated above the pituitary gland. This allows it to perform one of its main functions which is to regulate the flow of hormones to the pituitary gland. It also has other vital functions as:
Control centre for the autonomic nervous system
Appetite regulator
Body temperature regulator

Functions of the Cerebellum

The cerebellum governs fine movement and co-ordination. Patients when asked by a doctor to place a finger on their nose with both eyes shut, are being tested, along with other areas, on the function of the cerebellum.

Functions of the Brain Stem

The **midbrain** and **pons** are mostly concerned with the conduction of nerve impulses to and from the brain. The pons also conducts some impulses to and from the cerebellum. These areas also give rise to some of the 12 pairs of cranial nerves.

The **medulla oblongata** situated at the base of the brain stem joins with the pons at the top and the spinal cord beneath. As the medulla passes through the foramen magnum (the opening in the base of the skull) it becomes the spinal cord. The medulla contains many of the vital control centres of the body. It contains the controls for respiration, heart action, and the level of consciousness. It is also the centre which governs our reflex actions of: swallowing, blinking, coughing, sneezing, continence and vomiting.

Control of Continence. Remember that continence is governed by two controls involuntary and voluntary:

The **involuntary** reaction means that when the bladder contains a certain amount of urine the spincter is stimulated and by reflex control urine is passed. This is the condition with a baby until toilet trained. Toilet training means that continence has been brought under voluntary control. With **voluntary** control, although a certain amount of urine is in the bladder the spincter is again stimulated but this time the central nervous system takes control and urine is not passed until the right time and place are decided on. This situation of a dual control refers to the bowel as well as to the bladder.

It follows from this that a patient with some disturbance of consciousness is suffering from some disturbance in the function of the medulla oblongata. The medulla oblongata can be affected by damage or disease from the beginning of the illness or from conditions of the brain which may result in raised intracranial pressure, e.g., haemorrhage or brain swelling. Whatever the cause something is increasing the pressure within the skull. The only exit for swelling or misplaced brain tissue is downwards towards the medulla oblongata and the only opening from the skull — the foramen magnum. This creates pressure on the medulla and alters its function, it also causes displacement of the brain — herniation (Figure 44). Whether the effect on the medulla is initial or delayed the disturbances in its function are important because they require accurate nursing observation and nursing care to prevent serious complications. It is important for the nurse to identify the changes in the patient.

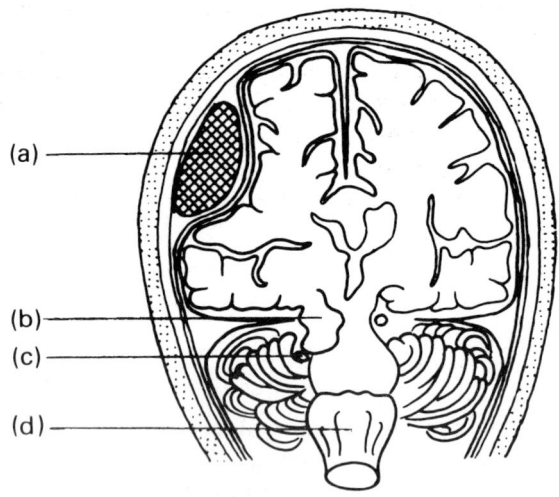

Figure 44 The result of increased intracranial pressure. A subdural haematoma (a), causes herniation of the cerebrum (b), displacement and pressure on the oculomotor nerve (c), and pressure on the medulla oblongata (d).

Causes

There are many different causes of unconsciousness which come about due to a disturbance in the brain cells, e.g., from a lack of blood, a change in blood concentration, irregularities within the chemical balance of the cells or a response to electrical stimuli. Here are a few of the causes:
  Accident — trauma
  Epilepsy — endocrine
  Intracranial ischaemia — infections, tumours
  Opiates — overdoses of gases, alcohol, drugs.
  Uraemia — metabolic disturbances, i.e., diabetes.

Determinants

It is important to determine the cause of unconsciousness as, although basic nursing care of the unconscious patient is the same, the medical management varies (Figure 45).

Means of determining cause of unconsciousness:
1 History from relatives, friends, witnesses or ambulance personnel.
2 General observation of the patient for trauma or obvious abnormality.
3 The unconscious patient will be unable to say whether there is any pain so observe the body closely for any obvious deformity, bruising or other injury.
4 The patient may smell of:
  Hay (sweet-like) — indicating acetone on the breath.
  Alcohol
  Vomit

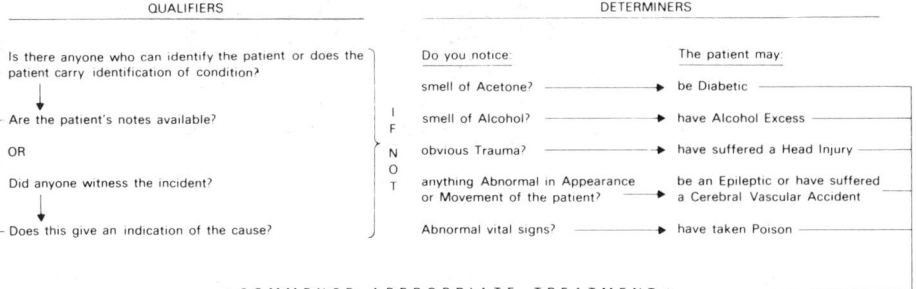

Figure 45 Steps towards determining the cause of unconciousness.

The Unconscious Patient

5 The patient may have an identification bracelet, necklace, or card which may indicate epilepsy or diabetes.
6 Blood tests. Normal blood glucose level is 3.9–5.6 mmol litre^{-1} and normal blood urea level is 2.9–8.9 mmol litre^{-1}.
Blood is also sent for toxicology testing. This will determine if poisons are present and the type and amount of substance in the blood.
7 Skull X-rays.
8 Urine samples. These can determine:
Glucose content in urine (normal — nil)
Toxic substance in urine — some poisons are excreted in the urine.

HEAD INJURIES

Head injuries involve any damage to the structure of the head. The structural layers of the head (figure 46) are the scalp, the skull, the meninges and the brain. The meninges are composed of 3 layers:
Dura mater — Outer 2 layers of dense fibrous tissue
Arachnoid — Middle layer of delicate serous membrane
Pia mater — Inner layer of fine vascular membrane which closely surrounds the brain
Injuries can be inflicted on any or all of these layers and may result in concussion and disturbance of consciousness.

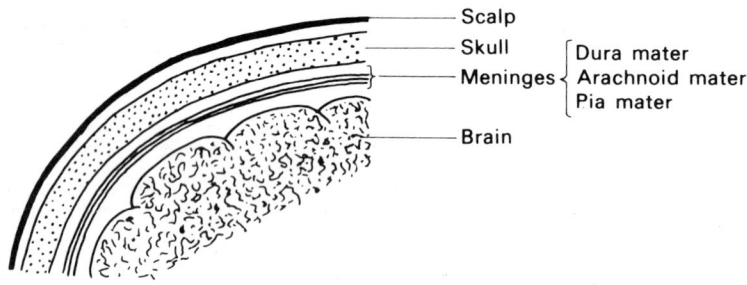

Figure 46 The structural layers of the head, protecting the brain, are all liable to injury.

Scalp. Injuries to the scalp include:
Contusion — bruising
Laceration — jagged cut
Puncture wound — deep cut
Avulsion — peeling off of skin

Skull. Injuries to the skull involve:
Bone injuries — fractures

Types of fractures:
Closed — bone broken but no skin wound communication with fracture
Compound — bone broken with a skin wound communication with fracture

Complications of fractures:
May involve meninges causing tearing and damage to blood vessels
May compress brain tissue
May damage brain tissue
May lead to infection if compound
A fractured base of skull may result in leakage of cerebrospinal fluid from the nose or ears causing an added complication of infection.

Meninges and Blood Vessels. Injury to the meninges can be caused by tearing.
If the blood vessels are involved then haemorrhage results.
The cerebrospinal fluid circulates between the arachnoid and pia mater and any haemorrhage into this space (the subarachnoid space) will be diagnosed by a lumbar puncture which involves the removal of cerebrospinal fluid for examination.

Brain and Blood Vessels. Brain tissue damage can be caused by: Violent movement of the brain which may then result in any condition from concussion to unconsciousness. It is believed this disturbance of consciousness either temporarily or permanently with or without amnesia is due to the disturbance by movement of the reticular formation in the brain stem.
Laceration of brain tissue may be due to tearing or violent movement or from sharp pointed objects such as a dart. This is

an example of a puncture wound which has more serious consequences leading to unconsciousness or death because of the tissue it has affected.

Haemorrhage can also be the result of disease or trauma to blood vessels within the brain.

Effects

The effects of a head injury can be divided into 2 categories: primary and secondary brain damage.

Primary brain damage is the injury that occurs at the time of the accident; it may be severe enough to be fatal.

Secondary brain damage results from complications of the primary injury. This includes such things as:
Haemorrhage
Swelling of the brain
Increased intracranial pressure
Infection

Treatment

The treatment of a patient with a head injury, therefore, involves:
  Minimizing the effects of the primary injury
  Preventing complications
The treatment falls into 2 categories: general and specific.

General

General treatment of a patient with a head injury involves:
1   General assessment and treatment (see Chapter 3).
2   Continual observation depending on the patient's condition; every 15 minutes if seriously ill. Observations to be reported are:
  Rising blood pressure — hypertension
  Slow pulse — bradycardia
  Changes in levels of consciousness
  Alterations in respiratory rate and depth
  Cerebrospinal fluid leakage from nose or ears
The first 4 points, if observed, indicate a rise in intracranial pressure.

Specific

Specific treatment of a patient with a head injury involves:

Intravenous infusion. An intravenous infusion will be used for the administration of drugs to reduce raised intracranial pressure. The drugs used will be:
Diuretic — frusemide (Lasix); mannitol
Anti-inflammatory — dexamethasone (a steroid)
Anticonvulsant — diazepam (Valium); phenobarbitone

Skull X-ray. A skull X-ray will be taken from different angles to determine the fracture (Figure 47).

Surgery. Surgery will be performed to make burr holes in the cranium to remove the blood causing pressure on the brain.

If the patient has a discharge from the nose or ears:
1   Test discharge for glucose and protein. Cerebrospinal fluid contains 2.8–4.2 mmol litre^{-1} of glucose and 0.15–0.45 g litre^{-1} of protein. If the fluid contains glucose and protein then it is cerebrospinal fluid and the patient must have a communicating fracture at the base of the skull.
2   Aseptically clean the nose or ears or both with sterile normal saline and cover the area with sterile gauze to help prevent infection.

Outcome

The outcome will depend on the severity of the head injury and the treatment needed. The patient will be admitted to hospital in the case of severe injuries, or discharged home if the injuries are minor.

Advice on Discharge

After the doctor has examined and assessed the patient's immediate condition, the patient may not require admission to hospital and will be discharged. However, serious complications may occur after the initial injury and careful observations are essential. These should be continued by a responsible adult for at least 24 hours after the patient has been discharged.

If any of the following symptoms occur then the patient should return to the hospital **immediately**.
   Blurred or double vision
   Unusual eye movements

Excessive restlessness
Confusion or slurred speech
Inability to rouse the patient
Weakness or paralysis of the arms or legs
Convulsions or abnormal movements of the arms or legs
Vomiting
Temperature over 38°C (100.47°F)

The patient should be advised for the next 48 hours to:
1 Eat a light diet.
2 Avoid alcoholic drinks.
3 **Not** take sedatives or sleeping pills.

Epilepsy

Epilepsy results from disordered electrical activity within the brain. The disturbance varies in area and size from patient to patient and it depends on the area as to how the condition manifests itself in a patient.

Electroencephalogram

An electroencephalogram (EEG) traces the amplification of electrical impulses within the brain. Normal readings show regular repeating of recorded tracings (waves). These waves (Figure 48a) will vary with various activities, e.g., awake or asleep.

An electroencephalogram is a means of diagnosing epilepsy. In a patient with epilepsy the conduction of the nerve impulses has become irregular so that not only does the patient's behaviour become disturbed but the EEG tracing also shows abnormalities (Figure 48b).

Causes

Epilepsy is not a disease but a disorder of the brain which may be due to many different causes. The causes of epilepsy vary from disturbances within the brain (intracranial) to disturbances in the body (extracranial).

Intracranial causes can arise from:
Trauma
Infection, e.g., meningitis
Tumours
Vascular disorders

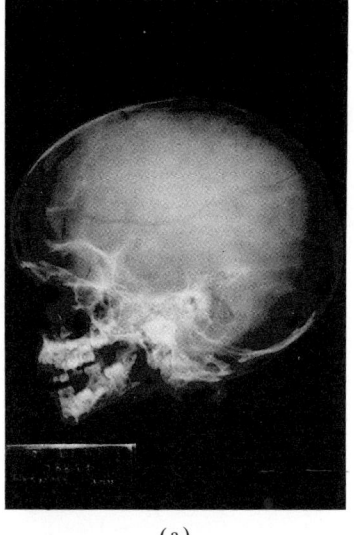

(a)

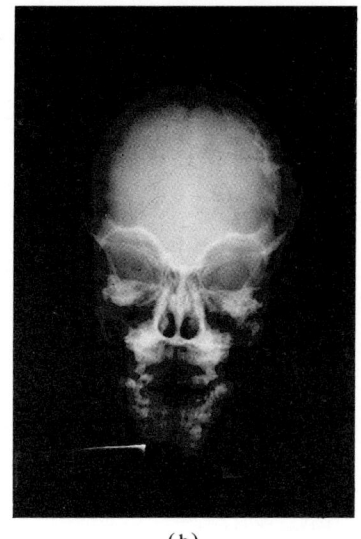

(b)

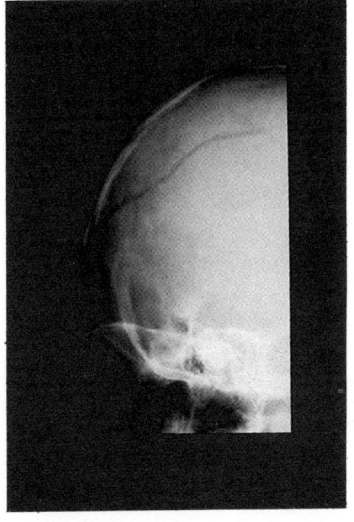

(c)

Figure 47 Slides of X-rays taken to determine the presence of a fracture of the skull: lateral view (a); frontal view (b); lateral posterior view (c). **Note** the difficulty of diagnosing the fracture and therefore the importance of X-rays taken from different angles.

Extracranial causes can be:
Electrolyte disturbances, e.g., can be produced by hyperventilation.
Toxic conditions, e.g., uraemia
Withdrawal from alcohol

Classification of Seizures

Epilepsy is classified depending on the effect displayed in the patient. Basically the classification is divided into 2 groups: partial or generalized seizures.

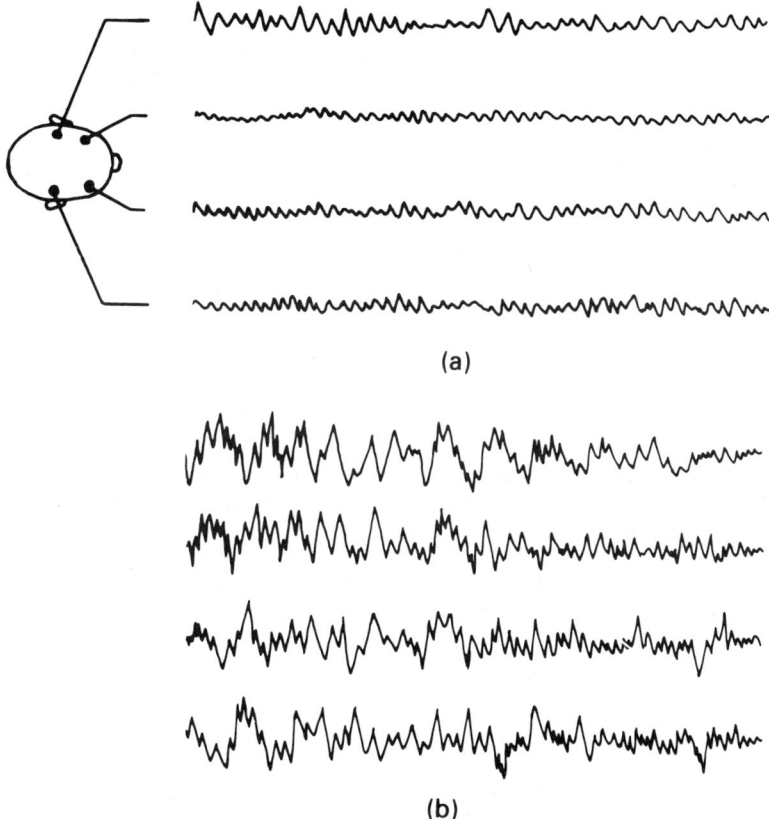

Figure 48 Electroencephalogram recordings: position of electrodes during recording and normal tracings (a); same electrode positions, showing the tracings from a patient with grand mal epilepsy (b).

Partial seizures involve only part of the body initially:
  Simple partial — Jacksonian
  Complex partial — involving the temporal lobe of the brain
Generalized seizures effect the whole body and are believed to start with disturbance in the reticular formation in the brain stem causing loss of consciousness.
  Simple absences — petit mal
  Tonic-clonic — grand mal
  Myoclonic

Partial Seizure

Jacksonian epilepsy is a form of epilepsy not often presented for treatment in the accident and emergency department. This epilepsy is a disturbance in the part of the brain which produces and co-ordinates movement. It produces twitching, muscular movement which may only effect a part of the body, e.g., the face or arm, but then may gradually spread throughout the body and produce the seizure which is most commonly seen in accident and emergency, the grand mal seizure.

Generalized Seizures

Petit Mal. Petit mal is a minor form of epilepsy. The patient suffers from periods of a loss of consciousness for a short time, usually a matter of seconds. For instance, most people are subject to slight losses of awareness but if fingers were snapped in front of them, they would react with a start and become aware of the noise. A person suffering from petit mal may not react to the noise initially. This type of patient does not usually attend an accident and emergency department because it is not an acute condition but he or she should be advised to see a doctor.

Epilepsy usually tends to start in childhood and it is often a school teacher who will discover that a child has petit mal epilepsy.

Grand Mal. Patients who suffer from grand mal epilepsy may be able to inform someone that they are about to have a seizure and they can then lie themselves down. The warning symptoms to the patient may be a strange smell or flashing lights. However, some patients have no warning at all.

The grand mal seizure has several distinct phases:
1 *Aura* (also part of a partial seizure) and serves as a warning and can include smells, laughter, flashing lights or déjà vu. Towards the end of this stage the patient will fall to the floor unconscious. The rapid escape of air forced from the lungs as the patient loses consciousness causes a sound known as 'the cry'.
2 *Tonic* when there is rigid contaction of all muscles. This may interfere with breathing and cause cyanosis. The jaw is clenched tightly shut and sputum may be present in the mouth. Normally this stage does not last long so that cyanosis or *apnoea* (lack of breathing) are not prolonged enough to cause serious complications.
3 *Clonic* when the muscles relax and the patient's muscles start to twitch and jerk. It is during this phase of muscle relaxation that the patient may be incontinent. Respiration may sound like grunts and the patient might now appear flushed.
4 *Postictal* when the patient regains consciousness and can present with any of the following:
Confusion
Drowsiness
Restlessness
Amnesia
Headache
The phase can last for several hours or even days. If the patient does not regain consciousness during the postictal stage there may be a reversion to the tonic phase with a recurrence of the seizure. This condition with a continual series of fits is known as *status epilepticus.*

Patient Care during Seizures

Postictal Phase. Patients are often admitted to the department following a grand mal seizure and are in the postictal phase. The nursing care during this stage comprises:
1 Careful observation of the patient until consciousness is regained completely. Be aware that the patient may revert to the tonic phase at any time. Also check to see if the patient has any self inflicted injury during the previous seizure, e.g., the patient's tongue or lips may have been bitten. Injuries may have been sustained when falling unconscious and there may be burns if the fall was near a fire.

2   Protection of the patient to prevent any harm being done. As the patient is often drowsy and confused, the patient needs to be nursed in an easily observed locale and in a semiprone position on a trolley with the safety rails up. Alternatively, the patient may be put in a wheelchair and securely fastened into the chair.
3   Reorientation of the patient. Remember that the last time the patient was conscious might have been when out shopping and the confusion may only result from the fact that the surroundings have altered totally.
4   Restraint of the patient if restless. The patient generally requires continual nursing if restlessness is the problem. This is done to protect the patient from self inflicted injury.

Aura Phase. If the patient actually falls to the floor in the aura stage in the department **give** the patient privacy. Screen the area where possible or lift the patient onto a trolley and into a cubicle. During the seizure:
1   Note the time the seizure started and when it finished.
2   Observe the patient and note whether the total body is affected or not. Note especially where the attack begins. Some patients although unconscious may only have movement of the facial muscles or a single limb.

Tonic Phase. During the tonic phase the most important priority of care is to maintain the airway. It is no longer advisable to put a wooden peg into the patient's mouth to prevent the tongue being bitten or obstructing the airway. The insertion of the wooden peg often meant that the patient's front teeth would be damaged because it is during the tonic phase that the jaw and teeth are clenched together, making it difficult to insert the wooden peg. In order to maintain the airway during this stage it is better to place the patient's head onto one side, or to place the thumbs or fingers behind the jaw bones and lift the jaw forward to ensure that the tongue stays forward (see Figure 6).

If the patient is producing sputum or vomitus then suction can be used to remove this. However, at this stage it is generally only possible to suction the mouth around the outside of the clenched teeth.

Clonic Phase. Remember that during the clonic phase the patient is still unconscious. It is essential to see that the patient is prevented from sustaining injury due to the jerking muscles and other involuntary movements. Make especially sure that the patient's head and limbs do not knock against any hard or sharp objects by placing pillows between the patient and the side rails of the trolley. This phase generally lasts for a few minutes; the patient moves from one phase to the next quickly.

Always ensure that someone stays with the patient during the seizure.

Rarely will a patient die during an epileptic seizure but the longer the seizure continues the more the patient becomes exhausted.

Drug Treatment

Drug treatment is used to control the seizure. There are several drugs of choice which are given intravenously initially:
Diazepam (Valium)
Phenobarbitone (Luminal, Gardenal) 50-200 mg. This dosage varies with the patient's age and it also depends on how the drug controls the patient's seizure.
Phenytoin sodium (Epanutin, Dilantin). This is given by slow intravenous injection, up to 250 mg at a rate not exceeding 50 mg per minute.
Before these drugs are given to control the seizure the doctor may take a blood sample to assess the present drug levels within the blood. Patients who are known to suffer from epileptic seizures are often controlled on regular dosages of antiepileptic drugs. However, insufficient or increased blood levels of the drug can produce seizures. It is important for the doctor to find out present drug levels so that it can be decided whether the drug therapy needs to alter. Alteration of drug therapy may require the patient to be admitted to hospital for observation and assessment.

Alternatively, upon regaining consciousness following a seizure the patient may be discharged home. **Ensure** that the patient is accompanied.

Convulsions

A *convulsion* is a sudden burst of electrical activity within the central nervous system which results in a disturbance in movement and a loss of consciousness. Convulsions in children before the age of five are generally associated with a rise in temperature.

Febrile Convulsion

With febrile convulsions a disease has resulted in a rise in temperature which leads to convulsions.

Treatment. Treatment of the child with a febrile convulsion:
1   Ensure that the airway is clear.
2   Prevent the child from self injury.
3   Record observations. It is important to take a rectal temperature to ensure the most accurate recording.

Procedures to Lower the Body Temperature. To lower the child's temperature:
1   Remove excess clothing. Leave the child covered by a sheet. Remember the parent or guardian will be extremely anxious so allow the accompanying adult to stay and assist in the undressing of the child. This will comfort and reassure both the distressed child and the parent or guardian.
2   Use a fan, if available, to cool the air.

Once the child has been seen by the doctor further measures may be taken to reduce the temperature:
   Administration of aspirin — this is an antipyretic which will
      reduce the temperature.
   Tepid sponging

Reduction of the temperature usually prevents further convulsions, however if the convulsion continues, drugs, e.g., intravenous diazepam (Valium) or intramuscular paraldehyde may be used to control the attack. Intramuscular paraldehyde will only be used if Valium has not controlled the attack.

Once the convulsion is controlled the doctor must ascertain the cause of the *pyrexia* (high temperature) and treat it accordingly.

The child will be admitted to hospital for observation, investigation and treatment.

Diabetes Mellitus

Diabetes mellitus is a metabolic disorder which can alter the conscious level. The disorder is caused by insufficient or complete absence of insulin production by the intra-alveolar cell islets, or islets of Langerhans, in the pancreas. Insulin is required for the transport of glucose into the cells and, if it is not produced, glucose accumulates in the blood. Glucose is produced for energy from the breakdown of carbohydrates and without this supply of energy, eventually the body has to begin to breakdown fats. This breakdown produces ketones and causes an acid base imbalance in the body which leads to the condition of *metabolic acidosis*. If diabetes mellitus is untreated and the patient develops *hyperglycaemia* (excess sugar in blood) this leads to *diabetic ketoacidosis*. Because of the disturbance of glucose and ketones the patient becomes unconscious, the condition generally known as *diabetic coma*.

Hyperglycaemia

Signs and Symptoms. The onset of hyperglycaemia is insidious. It can have developed over a period of days or even months. Often there is a history of a minor illness such as diarrhoea and vomiting or an infection. These conditions have either altered the body intake of carbohydrate or increased the body demand for glucose. The patient may not notice anything abnormal, or alternatively may complain of thirst, increasing tiredness, loss of weight, nocturia and increased urinary output *(polyuria)*. The polyuria can be severe enough to cause dehydration. The patient is often brought to accident and emergency unconscious or in a precoma state.

Observations. The nurse will observe that the patient is unconscious and has deep, noisy respirations — air hunger. Due to the metabolic acidosis of the condition the respiratory centre in the medulla oblongata is stimulated to try and rid the body of excess acid by expelling carbon dioxide which increases the respiratory rate. The presence of ketones in the body, produced by the breakdown of fat for energy, produces a sweet smell on the patient's breath, the smell of hay or acetone. The skin may show signs of dehydration (tenting) and the tongue and mouth appear dry and furred.

Tests. Urine tests reveal:
    Ketones — ketonuria
    Glucose — glucosuria

Blood sugar tests reveal an elevated blood glucose. The normal renal threshold is about 10 mmol litre^{-1}. However, in long-standing diabetes the renal threshold may have elevated to over 11.2 mmol litre^{-1} so that a diabetic patient may have an abnormally high blood glucose but the glucosuria is not so marked. That is why it is important to have accurate and regular recordings of both blood and urine tests. Unconscious patients will be catheterized to enable accurate and regular urine tests to be carried out.

Treatment. Primarily the treatment is to correct the excess glucose levels in the blood. This is done by the administration of insulin. Before insulin is administered the doctor will take a blood sample for serum glucose to get an accurate blood sugar level. The insulin can be given intravenously so that it starts to take effect within minutes or intramuscularly and starts to act within 10 to 20 minutes.

The insulin used for a diabetic coma is soluble because it starts to work quickly and works for a period of 4 to 6 hours. In a diabetic coma insulin is usually given initially by both intravenous and intramuscular routes. The reason for this being the necessity to control the diabetes but it must be done gradually otherwise a patient will change from a hyperglycaemic coma to a hypoglycaemic state. Then an intravenous infusion will be commenced. The solution used will depend on the patient's estimated blood sugar level from a dextrostix before the laboratory results of blood glucose are available. Insulin will also be administered depending on the patient's blood sugar level. A solution of normal saline will be commenced by infusion. The normal saline will correct the water balance of the dehydrated patient and so improve the condition. As the patient's blood sugar deceases the solution may be changed to:

Dextrose — saline (with a blood sugar level of 16.8 mmol litre^{-1})

5% dextrose (with a blood sugar level of 11.2 mmol litre^{-1})

It must be remembered that the patient may also require treatment for the precipitating disease whether it was a gastrointestinal disturbance or an infection.

As the treatment for a diabetic coma is the adjustment of blood glucose by insulin administration, it means that the patient is admitted to hospital for the condition to be stabilized.

The patient is unconscious but with medical and nursing care the condition should improve within the following 24 hours. If the patient has had previous gastric disturbance such as diarrhoea and vomiting which has precipitated the coma the serum electrolytes will be unbalanced. If this is the case potassium may be added to the intravenous infusion.

Importance of Potassium

Potassium is responsible for muscle activity. Cardiac muscle is especially susceptible to changes in potassium levels and the muscle is affected by an increase in potassium *(hyperkalaemia)* or, as in the case of diabetic coma, a decrease in potassium *(hypokalaemia)*. Both situations produce general muscle weakness and eventually can cause alteration in heart function leading to cardiac asystole (cardiac arrest).

Normal blood potassium levels are 3.9–5.6 mmol litre^{-1}.

Nursing Care

Nursing care will involve accurate urine tests usually taken every 2 hours, so it is necessary to catheterize the patient. Make sure that at each 2 hourly period fresh urine is withdrawn from the catheter.

The doctor will take 2-hourly blood samples so that insulin dosages can be adjusted accordingly.

Follow-up care of any diabetic patient involves educating the patient about the disease. Diabetic coma (diabetic keto-acidosis) is a serious condition which requires rapid treatment to prevent the ultimate complication of death. Now due to treatment with insulin less than 2 % of diabetic patients will die from diabetic ketoacidosis.

If the patient is a known diabetic and is being treated with subcutaneous injections of insulin then further problems can develop. As the glucose the body requires is obtained from carbohydrate metabolism, a known diabetic patient is given insulin according to the required carbohydrate intake. The balance between carbohydrates and insulin must be maintained. If the patient takes insulin but not carbohydrates in sufficient quantity then the insulin will still utilize the glucose in the blood for the cells, but the blood levels of glucose will then be depleted. This leads to the condition of hypoglycaemia and the patient can lapse into unconsciousness.

Recognition of a coma is important and the type of unconsciousness must be determined as there are different sequences requiring separate treatments.

Hypoglycaemia

Signs and Symptoms. The onset of hypoglycaemia is sudden and usually occurs several hours after an injection of insulin with a history of a missed meal. The patient can usually describe the condition as it develops. He or she will complain of feelings of weakness, hunger, palpitations, faintness, dizziness accompanied by perspiration and mental confusion. The patient may be extremely rational but can also be extremely restless, confused and aggressive or sometimes the patient appears to be drunk. If the cause of the patient's behaviour is difficult to understand remember that a patient suffering from hypoglycaemia will not smell of alcohol.

Observations. Nursing observations will show a pale, perspiring patient with tachycardia. This is because hypoglycaemia has promoted the secretion of adrenaline. The function of adrenaline is to release the glycogen stored in the liver so that it can be used as glucose by the body. However, adrenaline also increases the heart rate and so produces the tachycardia. It also creates a tremor in the patient.

Observations of urine generally are normal.

Observations of the blood sugar are altered — blood sugar is decreased. Normal blood glucose is 3.9 - 5.6 mmol litre^{-1}. A quick test used in the accident and emergency department is the dextrostix test to determine the approximate blood sugar level. In the case of hypoglycaemia it will be less than 3.9 mmol litre^{-1}.

Treatment. Treatment in the initial stage of hypoglycaemia can prevent unconsciousness. As the patient has the condition due to a low blood sugar rapid replacement of glucose can correct the situation. So, if the patient has a swallowing reflex, a glucose drink such as orange with sugar in it or, alternatively, sweets or chocolate can be given.

If the condition is not corrected the patient will lapse into unconsciousness due to lack of glucose to the brain cells. Diabetic patients are taught to be especially aware of the symptoms of hypoglycaemia because repeated attacks of hypoglycaemia may lead to permanent mental changes.

When the patient is unable to swallow due to confusion or unconsciousness then the treatment is by intravenous injection of 25 g of glucose. Within 10 minutes of the injection of glucose the patient should regain consciousness. As soon as the patient is conscious and has a swallowing reflex a meal can be given to the patient before being discharged home. This meal provides the necessary carbohydrate content that the patient needs for the balance of insulin and glucose to be maintained within the body.

It is advisable to make sure that the patient is collected by someone and is also being looked after at home.

The treatment of a patient with hypoglycaemia is normally quick and effective once the condition has been diagnosed and rarely does a patient have to be admitted to hospital.

CEREBRAL VASCULAR DISORDER

A cerebral vascular disorder means that something has happened to the blood supply to the brain tissue. The brain is supplied with blood via the arterial circle, the circle of Willis (Figure 49) which is formed from the two carotid arteries and the two vertebral arteries.

Alteration in Blood Supply

Alteration in the blood supply can be due to haemorrhage, thrombosis or embolism. Cerebral **haemorrhage** can be due to:
  Weakening or abnormality of blood vessels, e.g., aneurysm
  Injury especially to the meninges, bleeding can occur at any level.

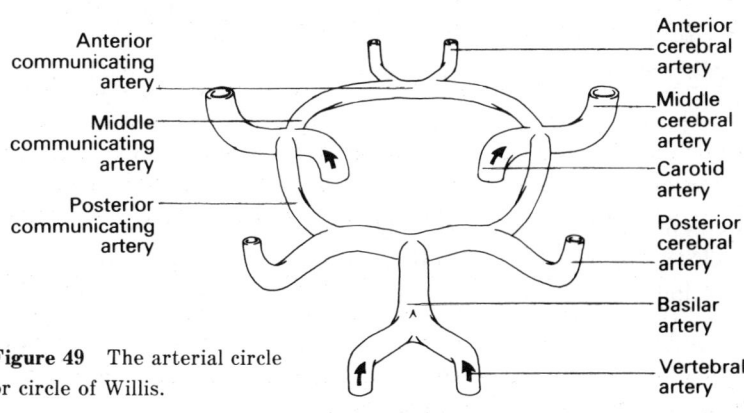

Figure 49 The arterial circle or circle of Willis.

Cerebral **thrombosis** is the gradual deposit of plaques on the inside of cerebral arteries until the blood supply is completely obstructed leading to death of brain tissue without the blood supply. This condition develops gradually.

Cerebral **embolism** is the sudden blockage of an artery at any point by a travelling emboli which totally obstructs the blood supply to the brain cells. The condition varies depending on the site and area affected. The patient may be paralysed due to damage to the area of the cerebrum, the frontal area, that controls movement. The patient may be unconscious due to the direct effect of alteration of blood supply to the medulla or from raised intracranial pressure, which has damaged the reticular formation within the brain stem. Raised intracranial pressure will arise from 2 causes:

1   The excess accumulation of blood in the cerebral cavity due to haemorrhage.
2   Swelling of the brain tissue itself due to irritation or damage.

Cerebral Vascular Accident

A cerebral vascular accident is better known as a stroke and is the most commonly encountered cerebral vascular disorder. The condition presents as an alteration in conscious level or an alteration in movement depending on the area and extent of brain tissue affected. The onset may be sudden or gradually progressive over a period of a few hours.

The patient is usually middle aged or elderly. Predisposing causes are hypertension or heart disease.

Cerebral vascular accident is only one example of an upper motor neurone disorder. This disorder means that the disease affects the motor neurone pathways from the frontal lobe of the cerebrum to the motor neurone in the anterior horn of the spinal cord.

Signs and Symptoms

Some of the features of an upper motor lesion include:
1   Exaggerated tendon reflex actions — the reflex arc is still functioning but there is no central nervous system control to make the reflex smooth and co-ordinated.
2   The limbs become spastic — the muscles are contracted as again the motor neurone of the reflex arc is holding the muscle

ready for action. The spasticity is usually unilateral affecting the side of the body opposite to the side of the brain which is affected. This is due to the fact that the nerve fibres cross over at the area known as the decussation in the medulla (Figure 50).
3   The Babinski's sign is positive — meaning that there is an abnormal reaction of the foot when a sharp instrument is stroked down the sole of the foot. Normal response is that the toe curls down (Figure 51a). Abnormal response is when the toe curls up (Figure 51b), this is present following a cerebral vascular accident and other disorders of the upper motor neurone tract.

These are observations the doctor will make during the examination of the patient.

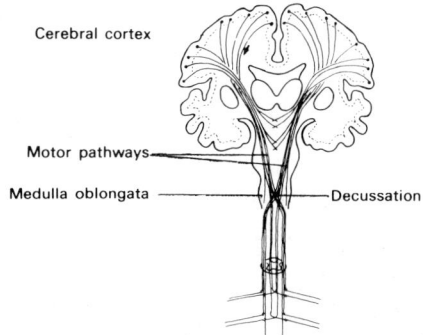

Figure 50   Upper motor neurone pathways showing the route of motor impulses (*arrow*) from the cerebral cortex through the spinal cord. The neurones cross over in the medulla oblongata area (decussation) resulting in the right side of the brain causing movement on the left side of the body.

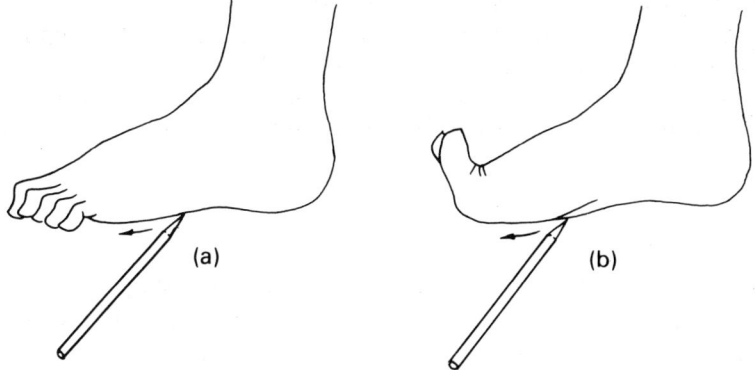

Figure 51   Reaction of the foot to a sharp object moving up its base: normal, the toes curl downwards (a) — a positive sign of upper motor neurone disease — Babinski's sign — when the toes curl upwards (b).

Determinants

The nurse can determine the patient's condition:
1 From the history. Any witness to the incident may state that the patient was well until sudden collapse or could not move or could not speak clearly.
2 By observing the patient:

The **facial appearance** will indicate whether one eye lid is drooping or one side of the mouth is sagging. If the patient is conscious test if the patient can smile and whether both sides of the mouth move equally.

The **limb movement** will indicate if any of the limbs are affected. The best way to test this is to ask the patient to grip both of your hands, then notice if the strength of the grip is equal in each side.

The **blood pressure** and **pulse** will indicate if there is a marked increase in these recordings.

The cause of a cerebral vascular accident is often hypertension so that recordings of a patient's blood pressure are often grossly elevated, e.g., 240/130 mmHg. Other conditions of unconsciousness do not cause such grossly elevated blood pressures from the initial stages.

The **state of consciousness** can vary tremendously; the patient can be deeply unconscious and unresponsive to any stimuli or may just have difficulty in speaking. If the history is linked with these observations the nurse can begin to understand the cause.

Treatment

If the patient is unconscious then treatment for an unconscious patient **must** be given (see p. 56).

The initial effects of a cerebral vascular accident may subside over a few days as the inflammation and oedema caused by tissue death decreases, so improvement in the condition of the patient may be possible. Because of this the treatment for a patient following a cerebral vascular accident is largely preservation. That is **maintaining** the vital functions.

In order to decrease the effects of the condition, drugs may be given to:

Decrease the amount of cerebral oedema.
Limit the size of the blood clot if the cause has been an embolism or thrombosis.

Drugs used are:
  Dexamethasone — an anti-inflammatory drug, corticosteroid.
  Heparin — an anticoagulant, will limit the formation of blood clots (emboli or thrombosis). It will not be administered if bleeding is suspected.

Patient Care

For patient care:
If the patient has vomited, it is essential to clear the airway to prevent inhalation.
If the patient has been incontinent, then clothing must be changed and the patient washed and dried carefully.
Following a cerebral vascular accident the patient requires admission to hospital.
Ensure that the next of kin is notified. However, remember this is a condition which usually affects the elderly so that the next of kin is often elderly. Before informing the next of kin about the condition of the patient, ascertain that there is someone else present if needed.

POISONING

Unfortunately poisoning is becoming one of the commonest conditions being seen in an accident and emergency department. It is also a condition which affects all age groups.
  A poison can be anything taken into the body in a sufficient quantity to cause a harmful effect to the body.
Routes by which poisons can enter the body:
  Mouth — as tablets or liquids.
  Respiratory tract — as gas, e.g., carbon monoxide
  Skin — in the form of insect bites or snake bites, or an injection
Due to the variety of poisons there are many effects, but poisoning can be a cause of unconsciousness.

Determinants

The nurse can determine the cause from:
1 History. The history can be provided by a relative, friend or

ambulance personnel, determined from the situation and often the fact that there is a note or empty bottle of tablets near the patient.

2 Age of the patient. Patients aged between fifteen and sixty with no other obvious cause of unconsciousness can be observed for signs of acute poisoning.

3 Blisters on skin especially in crevices. Some poisons, particularly barbiturates, cause skin blistering and are diagnostic signs of poisoning.

4 Needle marks in the skin related to blood vessels. This can indicate that the patient is injecting with intravenous drugs.

History

Information is needed to provide the history of the patient's condition.

1 *Which tablets or solution was taken.* As poisons can have so many different effects it is necessary to know what is being dealt with; the possible effects; and how to combat them.

2 *What amount was taken.* It is not always possible to get an accurate number or amount but an estimation can give an idea of the probable effects of the poison.

3 *Time when taken.* If the poison was taken by mouth it should remain in the stomach for 4–6 hours. This means that in some cases the poison can be removed from the stomach in this time. Aspirin remains in the stomach for a longer period, up to 24 hours, because it forms itself into a ball in the stomach. This means that in the early stages of an aspirin poisoning the total amount of the poison might not have been absorbed into the body, but over the following 24 hours the blood level and harmful effect of aspirin can increase.

4 *Whether taken with alcohol.* Alcohol accentuates the action of any poisons and so renders them more harmful to the body. Make sure that if there is a smell of alcohol the patient is not also suffering from an overdose of poison. This factor is not always easy to determine. The history may indicate that a poison has been taken with alcohol. Other indications may be skin blisters or a deteriorating level of consciousness. Blood samples for toxicology will definitely confirm whether a poison has been taken.

Treatment of Oral Poisons

Treatment of oral poisons depends on several factors:
1 Whether the patient is conscious or unconscious.
2 Which poison the patient has taken.
3 The effect the poison is producing in the patient.

Aims of treatment:
1 Neutralize the poison.
2 Eliminate the poison.

Poisons can be divided into 2 main groups, corrosive and noncorrosive poisons.

Corrosive poisons includes any tablet or substance which will cause burning, e.g., acids or clinitest tablets (used by diabetics to test their urine for the level of glucose). This group can be further subdivided into substances which are known as volatile corrosives. *Volatile corrosives* have fumes which cause problems when inhaled. In addition they are absorbed into the body in the presence of fatty substances as they pass through the digestive system.

Noncorrosive poisons do not burn and include all tablets which can normally be taken by mouth.

Corrosive Poisons

The treatment for corrosive poisoning involves neutralizing the poison and accelerating the movement within the gastrointestinal tract to rid the body of the poison. Because of the risk of burning in the mouth and oesophagus it is important that the patient does **not** vomit as this would subject the tissues to the burning substance twice.

Corrosive poisons are treated with the administration of milk, water or orange juice.

Volatile corrosives are treated with skimmed milk as this does not contain the fatty substances of ordinary milk which would accelerate the absorption of the poison.

If the patient complains of pain behind the sternum (substernal pain) when oral fluids are being given, the nurse must stop the oral fluids and notify the doctor immediately. The burning on ingestion of the poison has in this case caused ulceration or perforation of the oesophagus. This condition will require surgery.

Noncorrosive Poisons

The treatment for noncorrosive poisoning depends on the poison taken.

The conscious patient is treated in the first aid situation by being induced to vomit. This can be done by putting two fingers to the back of the patient's throat.

Once in hospital, the treatment can include either:

1 Administration of an emetic. An emetic such as ipecacuanha can be used. The usual dose is 30 ml. This is given with copious fluid to induce vomiting. Tepid fluids produce a better result. Water can be given or, in the case of children, orange juice is tolerated more easily. It is essential for the patient to co-operate during this procedure. Parents or guardian may be helpful in encouraging a child to drink the fluids and are often left with the child to ensure that the fluid is taken.

2 A gastric lavage.

Gastric Lavage

A gastric lavage is an unpleasant procedure for the patient and requires the patient's co-operation, if conscious. However, this procedure can be performed on both conscious and unconscious patients to remove the poison from the stomach and so prevent further absorption.

With an unconscious patient it is essential to protect the patient's airway so the patient must be seen by an anaesthetist and have an endotracheal tube put in position to maintain the airway. If an endotracheal tube has been passed, then an anaesthetist must remain in attendance during the gastric lavage procedure. The procedure is only performed within 4-6 hours of the poison being taken (except in the case of aspirin) because after this time the poison has passed further along the alimentary tract.

In some accident and emergency departments the doctor will perform a gastric lavage whereas in others, competent nursing staff perform the procedure.

Complication. Complications from the procedure are rare but can include:

Oesophageal trauma
Gastric bleeding

Water intoxication — due to the fact that the irrigated fluid is not returned but left in the patient's stomach.
Inhalation of gastric contents
To prevent inhalation:
1 Position patient correctly in a left lateral position.
2 Elevate the patient's feet to allow the gastric contents to flow down to the mouth.
3 Have suction equipment available.

To prevent these complications it is essential to follow the procedure.

Preparation. It is important to prepare the patient by explaining the method and to obtain co-operation to prevent a traumatic procedure.

The nurse can ensure correct positioning, by laying the patient on the left side with the left arm bent behind the back. This makes it easier for the nurse to hold the patient to prevent the stomach tube being pulled out once it has been inserted. For this reason the doctor or nurse must ensure that there is sufficient assistance or help before starting the procedure.
The minimum requirement of staff for the procedure is 3 people:
 One to restrain the patient and operate suction equipment.
 One to pass the stomach tube. This must be a doctor or a trained nurse.
 One to perform the lavage.
If restless or aggressive, it may take more than 3 people to restrain the patient.
Before procedure:
1 Position patient and elevate foot of trolley
2 Protect trolley with plastic drawsheet and incontinence pad.
3 Collect all equipment.
4 Place vomit bowl by patient in case vomiting takes place as the tube is passed or during the procedure.
5 Connect tubing and turn on suction
6 Make sure that you have enough help.

Procedure. To perform a gastric lavage:
1 Lubricate the stomach tube with lubricating jelly or water. Put the tube in the patient's mouth and ask the patient to swallow. As the patient swallows move tube smoothly and

quickly through mouth into the stomach.

2 Once the tube is in the stomach aspirate a small amount of the contents and test on Litmus paper to see if the tube is in position. If the tube is in place the blue litmus paper will turn pink.

3 The assisting nurse will connect the tubing and funnel to the stomach tube. Keep the funnel lower than the trolley and fill with the irrigating tap water. The funnel is then raised until all fluid has gone into the stomach.

4 Once the fluid has gone into the stomach the funnel is lowered to beneath the level of the trolley and placed over the bucket on the floor. Observe the fluid contents. If blood returns do not continue the procedure but inform the doctor.

5 From the first funnel of stomach contents take a specimen of fluid to be sent to the laboratory for analysis. Then empty the funnel contents into the bucket. Ensure that you are getting back the same amount of fluid that is being put into the stomach.

6 Continue the procedure until the stomach contents returned in the funnel are clear. Do **not** use more than 2 litres of water. If the return is not clear after using 2 litres the doctor will decide whether to continue.

7 At the end of the procedure disconnect the stomach tube from the funnel and tubing and slowly remove the gastric tube.

8 Make sure that the patient is left clean, dry and comfortable.

9 Turn off the suction apparatus and return the trolley to its original level.

Observations

Because of the number of effects poisons can have on various systems of the body it is vital for the nurse to observe the effects on the:

Respiratory system
Circulatory system
Nervous system

An increased heart rate may mean a lower blood pressure (hypotension) so that a patient may be in a condition of shock (see Chapter 3). Some drugs taken in excess directly cause hypotension, respiratory depression and alteration in conscious level, e.g., barbiturates, morphine.

Effects

Most systems of the body are affected by poisons in one way or another (Table 6). The symptoms which require treatment will depend on the poisons present. This is a quick reference to some of the common poisons and their effects on each system. The poisons which cause these effects are summarized as those poisons which:
    Increase (accelerate) the functioning of the system.
    Change the function of the system.
    Slow (depress) the system.

Symptoms and Treatment of Some Poisons

Ethyl Alcohol

The acceptable level of alcohol is less than 0.80 g litre^{-1} of plasma. This is the legal driving limit in Great Britain. Severe poisoning may involve as much as 3.00 g litre^{-1} of plasma.

Symptoms. Symptoms of ethyl alcohol poisoning include:
    Alteration in levels of consciousness from muscular inco-ordination, blurred vision, slurred speech, drowsiness to unconsciousness.
    Tachycardia
    Slow respirations
    Hypothermia

Treatment. In severe cases treatment would be with emetic drugs and a gastric lavage and removal of the poison by:
    Peritoneal dialysis
    Haemodialysis
The patient would be treated for the overall symptoms especially for respiratory and cardiac changes.

Antidote. The antidote for ethyl alcohol poisoning is fructose administered intravenously.

Bleach

The effect of bleach depends on which chemicals the manufacturers have used in its production.

Table 6 The effects of poisons on the systems of the body.

System	Accelerate	Change	Depress
Respiratory	Causing hyperventilation: Salicylates Carbon monoxide Iron	Causing pulmonary oedema: Carbon monoxide Causing dyspnoea: Paracetamol	Causing hypoventilation: Alcohol Barbiturates Morphine
Circulatory	Ethyl alcohol Carbon monoxide Paracetamol	Causing arrhythmias: Paracetamol Causing coagulation: Salicylates	Bleach Iron Causing hypotension: Barbiturates Morphine
Nervous	Leading to convulsions: Bleach Iron	Carbon monoxide Causing pin-point pupils: Morphine Causing tinnitus, deafness, blurred vision: Salicylates	Alcohol Barbiturates Laburnum seeds Morphine
Temperature regulation	Causing hyperpyrexia: Carbon monoxide Salicylates		Causing hypothermia: Ethyl alcohol Barbiturates Morphine Paracetamol

Table 6 cont.

System	Accelerate	Change	Depress
Gastrointestinal and metabolic function	Causing diarrhoea: Laburnum seeds	Causing nausea and vomiting: Alcohol Carbon monoxide Iron Laburnum seeds Paracetamol Salicylates Causing abdominal pain: Iron Laburnum seeds Salicylates Causing haematemesis and melaena: Carbon monoxide	Causing liver damage: Iron Paracetamol Causing hypoglycaemia: Paracetamol Salicylates Causing paralytic ileus: Barbiturates

Symptoms. Symptoms include:
- Irritation of the upper gastrointestinal tract
- Oedema of pharynx and larynx
- Nausea and vomiting
- Muscular twitching and convulsions
- Shock and cardiac arrest
- Acute renal failure

Treatment. Treatment would involve a gastric lavage because the bleach has a corrosive effect when in contact with the hydrochloric acid of the stomach.

Antidote. The antidote for bleach containing sodium hypochlorite is *sodium thiosulphate* which is given either directly or intravenously into the stomach. For bleach containing oxalic acid, *calcium lactate* is given with lavage fluid or left in the stomach, or *calcium gluconate* is given intravenously.

Barbiturates

Symptoms. Symptoms of barbiturate poisoning include:
- Alteration in levels of consciousness leading to coma.
- Depression of respiratory function
- Hypothermia
- Alteration in the gastrointestinal system causing, in severe cases, a paralytic ileus.
- Skin blisters
- Alteration in the circulatory system, peripheral vasodilation.
- Hypotension
- Shock

Treatment. Treatment would include:
- Emetic drugs — if the patient is conscious.
- Gastric lavage — if the patient is unconscious, an endotracheal tube must be in place.

In addition, the patient would receive overall treatment for accompanying symptoms of shock, alterations in respiratory function and hypothermia.

Carbon Monoxide

Symptoms. Symptoms of carbon monoxide poisoning include:

Alteration in levels of consciousness from agitation to mental confusion to coma.
Pyrexia
Damage to the central nervous system which may result in paralysis, Parkinsonism or personality changes.
Changes in circulatory function, tachycardia
Hypotension leading to the condition of shock
Myocardial ischaemia and infarction
Respiratory changes due to hypoxia — hyperventilation, pulmonary oedema, respiratory failure.

As the carbon monoxide attaches itself to the haemoglobin in the erthrocytes and displaces oxygen, it forms carboxyhaemoglobin which in severe cases gives the patient's skin and mucous membranes a pink colour. Alternatively the patient may be pale in appearance. Skin blistering may also be present. There may be nausea and vomiting, incontinence of faeces, haematemesis and melaena.

Treatment. Treatment involves removal of the patient from the poisonous atmosphere. Oxygen is administered and conditions such as pulmonary oedema and myocardial infarction are treated.

Iron

Symptoms. Symptoms of iron poisoning include:
   Nausea and vomiting
   Abdominal pain
   Deep and rapid respirations
   Changes in conscious level
   Convulsions
   Circulation failure
   Liver damage
   Acute renal failure

Treatment. For treatment following iron poisoning, a patient is always admitted to hospital for a gastric lavage and is kept in hospital for 12–24 hours for observation of the effects of the poison. Generally, it is children who are admitted with this type of poisoning.
A gastric lavage is used due to the irritant effect of the iron once it is in the stomach.

Antidote. Desferrioxamine B mesylate is given in one of three ways:
   Intramuscular injection
   Left in the stomach following gastric lavage
   Intravenous injection

Laburnum Seeds

Symptoms. Symptoms of laburnum seed poisoning include:
   Burning of the mouth and throat
   Nausea and vomiting
   Abdominal pains
   Diarrhoea
   Drowsiness, inco-ordination
   Confusion, twitching and coma

Treatment. Treatment involves a gastric lavage and the patient is treated according to the symptoms.

Morphine

Symptoms. With morphine and other controlled drugs, the symptoms of poisoning include:
   Alteration in levels of consciousness leading to unconsciousness
   Respiratory depression
   Pin-point pupils
   Hypotension
   Hypothermia

Treatment. The effects on the respiratory system are treated along with the treatment of the other symptoms.

Antidote. The antidote for morphine poisoning is *naloxone hydrochloride* (Narcan) which is a respiratory stimulant. It may also make the patient extremely restless so it is important to protect the patient from self-inflicted injury after the antidote is administered.

Paracetamol

Symptoms. The immediate effects of paracetamol poisoning are

usually mild for the first 24-hours and include:
  Nausea and vomiting
  Pallor and perspiration
However, the patient may be suffering from the effects of the poison on the central nervous system. This may produce unconsciousness.
Later effects include:
  Hypothermia
  Hypoglycaemia
  Metabolic acidosis
  Respiratory problems, e.g., dyspnoea
  Hypotension
  Tachycardia
  Cardiac arrhythmias
  Renal and hepatic failure

Treatment. Treatment depends on the level of consciousness and will involve emesis or a gastric lavage. This treatment must be carried out within 4 - 6 hours of ingestion.
The patient must also be treated according to the symptoms.

Antidote. The antidotes given are:
  Methionine — orally
  Cysteamine — intravenously
  Acetylcysteine — intravenously

Salicylates

Symptoms. Symptoms of salicylate poisoning include:
Alteration in respiratory function:
  Hyperventilation — causing alteration in the acid base balance of the body *(respiratory alkalosis)*
  Pulmonary oedema
Dehydration due to:
  Abdominal pain and vomiting
  Hypokalaemia
  Hypothermia with perspiring
Other effects produced are:
  Restlessness
  Ringing in the ears *(tinnitus)*
  Deafness
  Blurred vision

Hypoglycaemia
Hypothrombinaemia
Acute renal failure

Treatment. Treatment can involve the use of emetic drugs and a gastric lavage. A gastric lavage can be carried out up to 24-hours after ingestion as this poison tends to form into a ball in the stomach. The patient will be treated for electrolyte and metabolic disturbances (see p. 47).

Remove poison by:
Forced alkaline diuresis
Haemodialysis
Charcoal haemoperfusion

To treat poisoning correctly it is essential to ascertain the type of poison. Poison centres have been set up around the United Kingdom and provide a 24-hour service, supplying information on the accurate treatment of poisons. These centres are in London, Belfast, Cardiff, Edinburgh and Dublin, Eire.

REVISION OBJECTIVES

1 Define the term unconsciousness and identify vital factors in patient care.
2 Describe and illustrate the structure and function of the central nervous system.
3 Identify and annotate the causes of unconsciousness.
4 Detail the structures of the head and list the various injuries which can occur.
5 Describe the treatment of a patient following head injury.
6 Describe the condition of epilepsy, detailing the signs, symptoms, nursing care and medical treatment.
7 Describe a febrile convulsion and the methods of patient care.
8 Describe the condition of diabetes. Identify and treat hypoglycaemic and hyperglycaemic comas.
9 Outline the normal and abnormal physiology related to a cerebral vascular disorder and describe the signs, symptoms and treatment.
10 List the effects of poisons on the body and describe the treatment for and the effects of common poisons on the systems of the body.

9
Bone and Soft Tissue Trauma and Plastering

TRAUMA

Trauma can be defined as an accidental physical injury which causes damage to the body structure or alters the body function. The types of injury can involve various systems of the body:
  Integumentary skin (see Chapter 4)
  Skeletal (see p.211)
  Neurological (see Chapter 8)
  Respiratory
  Cardiovascular
  Digestive involving abdominal organs, especially the spleen and liver
  Renal
  Reproductive

By knowing the normal anatomy and physiology of the various systems it is possible to observe the changes which may occur due to injury. The related locations and effects of injury are shown in Table 7. These injuries will be dealt with in isolation; it must be remembered that some patients receive multiple injuries. The nurse must be alert to the most serious condition of the patient.

Table 7 Related locations and effects of injuries.

Location of injury	Effect of injury
Head, face	Lacerations, contusions, fracture.
Chest	Rib fractures; flail chest, respiratory disturbance; pneumothorax; haemothorax.
Abdomen	Rupture of spleen, kidneys, ureters.
Hips, pelvis	Fractures; rupture of bladder, damage to the urethra or reproductive organs.
Arms	Fractures; dislocation of shoulder.
Legs	Fractures; hip, femur, fibula, tibia, ankle.

Initial Care

The initial care, of any patient who enters accident and emergency following trauma, is to:
1 Assess the patient (see Chapter 3).
2 Determine priorities according to assessment.
3 Commence any emergency resuscitation.
4 Treat condition as necessary.

HEAD AND FACE INJURIES

With head and face injuries the main considerations are:
The **alterations** in the function of the central nervous system may result in the patient being semiconscious or unconscious (see Chapter 8).
The **obstruction** of the airway. In these injuries obstruction of the airway may come from a variety of sources:
   Teeth which have been loosened by the injury and swallowed.
   Dentures may also be dislodged and cause obstruction to the airway.
   Fracture of the bones forming the upper airway moving them out of position so that the airway is blocked.
   Haemorrhage from the injury in the upper respiratory tract.
   Loss of the swallowing reflex due to disturbance of the functioning of the medulla oblongata in the brain stem so that the patient's tongue blocks the airway.
If the airway is obstructed then this must be cleared by suction or removal of the obstructing matter (see Chapter 3).

Remember:
1 If the obstruction is due to excessive bleeding (haemorrhage) the patient will be suffering from shock (see Chapter 3).
2 Due to the obstruction the patient may suffer a lack of oxygen (hypoxia) so prepare the oxygen equipment for use.

Psychological Care

Patients with facial injuries require reassurance and careful explanations. They cannot see the result of the injury to their face and can only imagine the change, this often being based on the amount of pain being suffered and probably the taste of blood.

The only face the patient may see (if the eyes are not damaged) is that of the person caring for him or her — maintain a calm caring expression and control registering any facial reactions of shock. Talk to the patient but remember that the patient might have difficulty in speaking so phrase your questions for single answers.

Cleaning the patient's head or face may drastically alter the initial extent of the appearance of the injury. Once the patient's face has been cleaned with an aseptic solution (Savlon) then, if it has not been too distorted by the injury, it is advisable to allow the patient a mirror to quell the anxiety.

If the patient has received both head and facial injuries, treatment is generally conservative until the patient can be assessed fully with regard to the functioning of the central nervous system. This may mean that the patient may wait several days before a fractured jaw (mandible) is repaired surgically. However in cases of injury to the eye, such as when there are several glass fragments embedded in the eye, surgery will be carried out immediately to remove the fragments even if the patient has a head injury.

Do **not** give the patient with head or face injuries anything to drink before asking the doctor. If the patient has had bleeding into the mouth nursing care to the mouth is important. Check with the doctor before giving mouth care. A normal saline mouth wash is refreshing and clears the blood from the mouth.

CHEST INJURIES

Injuries to the chest can involve the heart and the lungs. Both of these organs are protected within the thoracic cavity by twelve pairs of ribs.

Heart

Injuries to the heart are serious due to the function and importance of the heart. As the heart is well protected by the ribs and the lungs, injuries are relatively rare.

Causes

Injuries can be caused by:

Stab wounds — directly penetrating part of the heart structure.

Direct blows — the apex of the heart (the point of the ventricles) is situated between the fifth and sixth rib towards the left side of the thoracic cavity. A direct blow to this area may result in bruising and bleeding of the blood vessels of the heart. Direct blows may come from blunt objects such as the steering wheel of a car.

Pierced by a bone — the heart may be pierced by a fractured bone, especially the sternum.

Bullet wounds

Signs and Symptoms

Injury to the heart results in:
Alteration of heart action — depending on the location and extent of damage.
   Haemorrhage leading to hypovolaemic shock.
   Ineffective heart action leading to cardiogenic shock.
   Absence of heart action (see Chapter 5).
In all these instances the patient may develop the signs and symptoms of shock. The alteration in heart action may also lead to cardiac arrhythmias.

Treatment

Treatment consists of maintaining an adequate heart function. This may involve:
1   Resuscitation.
2   Thoracic surgery. If the patient has an area within the heart which is bleeding then the chest is opened, the area located and the bleeding vessel cauterized or tied off. Likewise if the patient has a direct opening into the heart from a stab wound or gunshot wound then surgery is required to close that opening. The decision to perform surgery **must** be made immediately and carried out as quickly as possible.

The normal function of the heart is to pump blood to the brain and the body. To do this the heart pumps approximately 72 times a minute and pumps out 720 ml of blood each time, so that approximately 5 litres of blood flow through the heart each minute. An opening into the heart would result in the approximate loss of 2.5 litres of blood each minute. A loss of 3 litres of blood results in irreversible changes in the body due to hypovolaemia.

3 Rapid replacement of blood loss. This may be done with plasma initially until the correct blood group has been matched for the patient.

4 Oxygen therapy. Due to the loss of blood and consequent lack of oxygen to the tissues the patient will also require oxygen therapy.

5 Removal of blood by aspiration. If the bleeding has occurred into the pericardium this is known as a pericardial effusion and the blood may be removed by aspiration. The pericardium is composed of 2 layers:

The visceral layer on the outside.
The parietal layer lining the heart.

Bleeding or accummulation of fluid between these 2 layers causes a condition of cardiac embarrassment, *cardiac tamponade*, meaning that the heart cannot expand sufficiently when receiving blood, so that blood is unable to enter the heart effectively. The blood then begins to accumulate in the blood vessels of the lungs and in the general circulation. Once the area of bleeding has been located which will be demonstrated on X-ray then a cardiac needle may be inserted into the pericardial space and the fluid aspirated.

Injuries to the Lungs

Injuries to the lungs that allow air to enter abnormally into the lungs cause respiratory problems. The lungs are enclosed within the thoracic cavity and although the lungs contain air, the air is only allowed to enter and leave the lungs by the passage ways of the respiratory tract.

Causes

Injuries can be caused by:
   Direct blows to the chest from a blunt instrument
   Stab wounds to the chest
   Gun shot wounds
   Rib injuries
   Obstructed airway

The injuries alter the respiratory function by interfering with the mechanics of respiration (see p. 133).

Treatment

Treatment consists of maintaining an adequate respiratory function:
1 Clear the airway.
2 Observe respirations, noting rate, depth and rhythm, and if there is equal movement on both sides of the chest.
3 Observe the presence or effects of a cough.
4 Collect sputum. Damage to the lung tissue may produce bleeding so the patient will cough up blood *(haemoptysis)*. The nurse must be accurate in distinguishing between a haemoptysis and a *haematemesis* (the vomiting of blood). Both conditions require totally different treatment.
5 Maintain adequate lung ventilation.

Alteration in Inspiration

If the lungs have been injured then inspiration can be altered. Inspiration is the mechanical function of the rib cage and to allow air to enter the lungs the rib cage moves up and out and the diaphragm flattens. This makes the pressure within the lungs decrease and allows atmospheric air to enter.

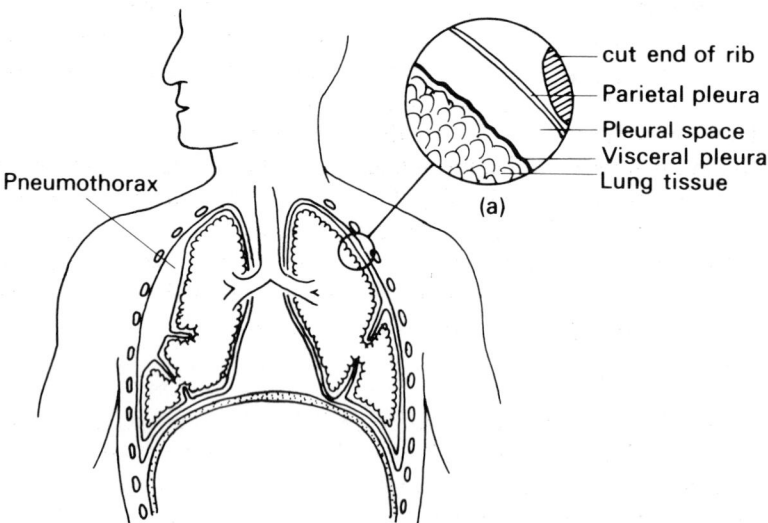

Figure 52   The chest cavity with a pneumothorax (air between the two pleural layers) in the right lung; detailed enlargement of a section through the chest cavity (a).

If there is injury to the lungs this may mean:

Air has entered the lungs from other sources and accumulated in the pleural space. This is the area between the two layers of pleura, the parietal and visceral which cover the lungs. This accumulation of air is known as a pneumothorax (Figure 52).

A blood vessel is damaged and there may be bleeding into the pleural space producing a haemothorax.

In either case the result is a decrease in the expansion of the affected lung and the affected lung begins to collapse.

Pneumothorax and Haemothorax

Signs and Symptoms. The signs and symptoms for a pneumothorax or haemothorax should involve a history of the incident.

However, a pneumothorax can develop from other causes not involved with trauma. This condition is known as a spontaneous pneumothorax when the patient's alveoli suddenly burst and instead of air entering the pleural space from without, air enters the pleural space from the lungs. This cause may be from chronic chest conditions or idiopathic.

There may be external signs of trauma:

Bruising.

A **puncture wound** resulting from a sharp point instrument or a bullet. If a puncture wound is located then it must be cleaned aseptically and covered with an airtight dressing to prevent further air entering the pleural space.

Deformity of the ribs can be due to fractures.

Subcutaneous emphysema which is another indication of chest injury occurs occasionally. This means that air has escaped from the lungs into the tissues and can spread to other parts of the body. Subcutaneous emphysema is observed by a crackling of the skin when it is touched. Once the cause of the air escaping is treated the subcutaneous emphysema gradually resolves.

Other signs may include: pain, especially on respiration causing dyspnoea. Pain will be localized to the area of injury and increase on forced inspiration. Consequently the patient's respiration will be shallow to limit the movement of the chest wall. Analgesia may be administered depending on the neurological condition of the patient.

As the patient's respirations are shallow there is generally an increase in the rate in order to obtain the necessary oxygen from the air.

If there is a deficiency in the amount of oxygen entering the lungs then the patient may appear cyanosed and require the administration of oxygen. Oxygen in this case may be given by nasal spectacles or via a mask.

Patients who develop the condition known as a *tension pneumothorax* appear extremely anxious, cyanosed and complain of dyspnoea. This is because the air has entered the pleural space from the lung and has created a high pressure as the air cannot return to the lungs. This causes severe tension within the pleural space and inhibits both the functions of the heart and the lungs. A tension pneumothorax is an emergency situation which requires **immediate** relief of the pressure.

Treatment. The aim of treatment is to remove the air or blood from the pleural space. It is necessary to find out the location of the pneumothorax or haemothorax and this is done with a chest X-ray.

Depending on the patient's condition it may also be necessary to take arterial blood samples for blood gases to find out the oxygen and carbon dioxide content of the blood (see Chapter 3).

To remove the air or blood from the pleural space a drainage tube (chest tube) is inserted. The procedure can be carried out under a local or a general anaesthetic by a doctor and may be carried out in the accident and emergency department.

A **local anaesthetic** is usually used in the case of a spontaneous pneumothorax. Following a chest X-ray the chest tube is inserted into the pleural space shown to contain air (Figure 53).

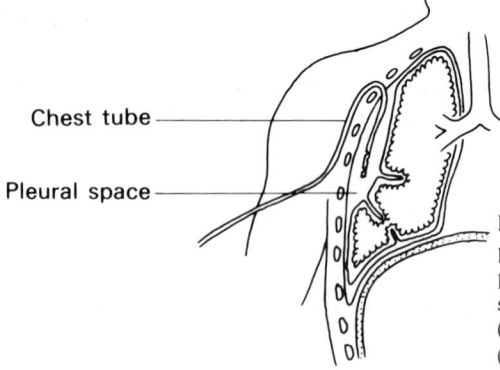

Figure 53 Chest tube in place between the two pleural layers. The pleural space can be created by air (pneumothorax) or blood (haemothorax).

As the patient is awake during the procedure it is important to explain the procedure and to reassure the patient throughout.

A **general anaesthetic** is used in the case of some injuries. The chest is opened surgically (thoracotomy) so that possible internal injury may be seen. This is especially needed in the case of a haemothorax where the damaged vessel may need to be located and the bleeding controlled. However, a thoracotomy is not always performed in instances of traumatic injury, and the chest tube may be inserted. In either case the patient will require admission to hospital.

When the chest tube is in position the patient may be nursed in a semirecumbent position or upright depending on observations of blood pressure and other injuries.

Care of the chest drain
1 It is essential that the chest drain is airtight, so it must be connected to either an underwater seal drainage system or a Heimlich flutter valve and drainage bag.
2 With a haemothorax it is vital to observe the amount of blood that is draining through the chest tube.

Conclusions

Treat as a **priority** the patient with injuries to the lungs:
1 Reassure. It is frightening to have dyspnoea.
2 Position. Upright or semirecumbent.
3 Seal any opening into the pleural space.
4 Administer oxygen if necessary.
5 Give analgesia if required. Once the patient has the chest tube in there may be reluctance to inhale deeply because this causes pain. Encourage the patient to breathe normally to enable expansion of the lung and prevent a chest infection.

Other respiratory disorders such as Cheyne-Stokes respirations are due to a disturbance in the medulla oblongata (see Chapter 8).

ABDOMINAL INJURIES

To understand the consequence of abdominal injuries it is important to know the contents of the abdominal cavity (Figure 54).

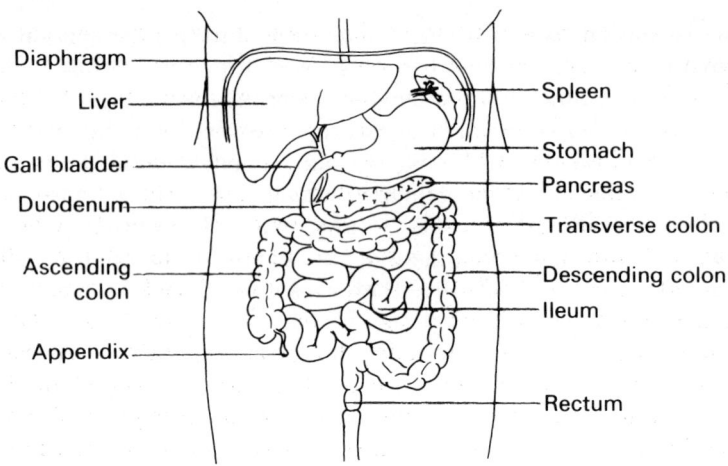

Figure 54 The abdominal contents. All organs and blood vessels are liable to injury.

Abdominal injuries can involve:

Tearing (rupture) of the organs within the abdominal cavity, e.g., spleen, liver, kidneys.

Direct damage to blood vessels of the abdomen, e.g., aorta, mesenteric, inferior vena cava, portal vein.

Bruising of the gastrointestinal tract. This bruising may result in a disturbance of function due to nerve involvement and cause a paralytic ileus.

Penetration of the gastrointestinal tract. This will result in the leakage of its contents into the peritoneal cavity causing peritonitis.

Causes

Injuries to the abdominal cavity can be caused by direct or penetrating blows.

A **direct blow** with a blunt instrument. There are a variety of causes such as a clenched fist, the steering wheel on a car, a stick or a crush injury.

A **penetrating blow** with a sharp instrument such as a knife or bullet. The extent and severity of a bullet wound depends on the weapon used. If the weapon used is a low velocity type, the bullet will pass through soft tissue injuring tissue in its direct path. A bullet from a high velocity weapon creates additional damage because as it passes through the tissue it creates a temporary cavity and also creates a force which can destroy tissue not directly in its path; so that a bone, although not directly hit, may be fractured. The easier the tissue is to pierce the less traumatic an effect the bullet will have. Bone, liver and spleen tissue being more condensed receive more damage from the force of the bullet. The temporary cavity formed by the passage of the bullet can pull into it external fragements of dirt. Therefore a bullet wound from a high velocity weapon is considered contaminated and requires aseptic cleaning. It must be remembered that a bullet travels either through the body or within the body. Therefore, it is important to locate the entrance wound and the exit wound if any in an attempt to locate the possible position of the bullet. A patient has been seen with a bullet wound in the right, mid-abdominal region and on X-ray the bullet has been seen to be lodged in between the patient's second and third lumbar vertebrae.

Patient Assessment

Assess the patient according to priorities. Regular observations must be made.

In many injuries to the abdomen the diagnosis is a suspected internal haemorrhage from a ruptured organ. Due to the fact that the spleen, liver and kidneys are all highly vascular organs, tearing or any damage to the organ is going to cause bleeding. This is internal haemorrhage. The patient may present with the signs and symptoms of shock, and will appear cold, clammy and anxious. Observations will show a low blood pressure and a rapid pulse. Treatment will depend on observations indicating the severity of the shock. Regular observations every 15 minutes will show if the internal haemorrhage is subsiding. This is important as surgery may only be carried out in deteriorating conditions or as a life-saving attempt.

Observations include:
1 Blood pressure
2 Pulse
3 Respirations. Pressure within the upper abdominal cavity will disturb the functioning of the diaphragm. Also some injuries may include both the thoracic and abdominal cavities.
4 Neurological state

5 Pain. It is important to assess the amount and type of pain the patient is experiencing. Abdominal pain can cause a tightening of the abdominal muscles known as guarding and the abdomen becomes rigid and board-like. Increasing pain would indicate an abdominal condition which requires exploratory surgery.

6 Girth measurement. The doctor will measure the patient's abdomen approximately at the level of the umbilicus. The exact area measured should then be marked on the patient by the doctor. This will ensure that a consistent recording is taken every 15 minutes.

The girth measurement is taken to assess whether the abdomen is distending due to:

Excessive bleeding

Obstruction of the bowel

Inflammatory condition of the bowel caused by perforation of bowel contents.

It is by taking observations and girth measurements that the surgeon will decide on the immediacy of an operation.

In the case of a suspected ruptured kidney urine tests are carried out. The patient may be catheterized and the urine tested for blood. Decreasing levels of haematuria mean that the bleeding within the kidney is being controlled whereas constant or increasing levels of haematuria and deteriorating observations require surgery.

Patient Care

Following abdominal injury the patient is either taken straight to theatre, in which case it is the responsibility of the nurse in the accident and emergency department to prepare the patient for an operation, or admitted to a surgical ward for observation.

In all cases the patient must be reassured. The necessity for the hospital admission was unexpected and may be completely inconvenient for the patient. Notify the next of kin, by telephone or police message, and make arrangements for a relative or friend to visit when suitable for the patient.

Treatment

To treat the condition of shock:

1 If blood pressure is not decreased, place in a semirecumbent

position. This is important especially in cases of gastrointestinal perforation, in order to keep the bowel contents which have entered the peritoneal cavity away from the liver or the diaphragm. Complications of liver abscesses or respiratory embarrassment (compression of the diaphragm) may result if contents are allowed to move freely around the peritoneal cavity.

2   A patient with hypotension must be nursed in the recumbent position.
3   Rest the patient's gastrointestinal tract by:
Keeping the patient nil by mouth.
Passing a nasogastric tube and connecting it to free drainage or aspirating it hourly. Remember to record the amount of aspirate and observe the type of aspirate.
4   Prepare an intravenous infusion for the doctor to commence which depending on the severity of shock may contain plasma, blood or artificial blood substitute (Haemaccel). Blood samples must be taken for cross matching before blood substitutes are infused.
5   Administer analgesia if ordered by the doctor.

Laparotomy

The operation to be performed in the first instance is a laparotomy and the consent of the patient, if over 16, must first be obtained before the operation is commenced. If the patient is under 16 see Chapter 2.

A *laparotomy* is an excision through the abdominal wall carried out for the purpose of exploring the abdominal contents and determining and correcting the result of the injury.

A **ruptured liver** can be treated by oversewing the edges or by a partial removal.

A **ruptured spleen** can be removed entirely (*splenectomy*).

With a **ruptured kidney,** the surgeon will attempt to retain as much of the organ as possible due to its essential functions. A partial nephrectomy may be carried out or in the case of a severe rupture a total nephrectomy. Before a total nephrectomy is performed the surgeon will ensure that there is another kidney present and that it is functioning adequately. To ensure this an intravenous pyelogram will be required.

LOWER ABDOMINAL INJURIES

The contents of the lower abdomen (Figure 55) are surrounded and protected in parts by the bones of the pelvic girdle. The contents are liable to injury from the same sources as the upper abdomen. However, pelvic injuries are often sustained as complications of injury to the bones (fracture) of the pelvis.

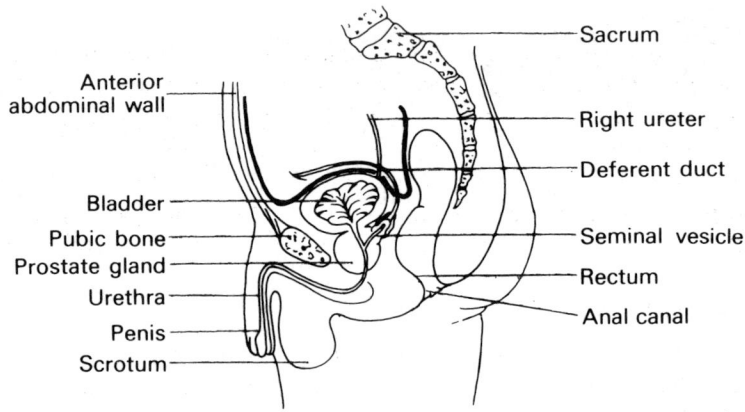

Figure 55a The male pelvic contents.

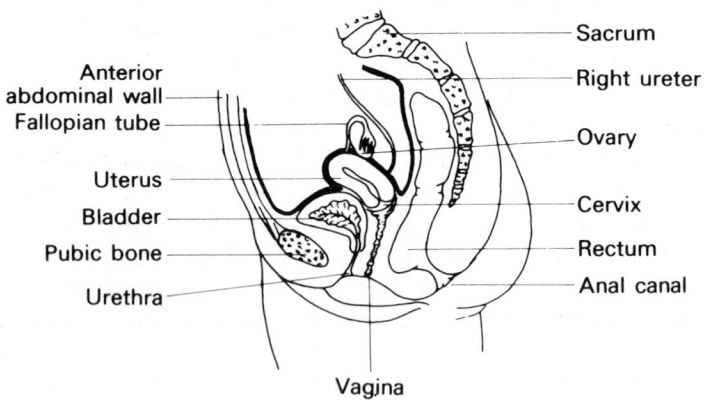

Figure 55b The female pelvic contents.

Signs and Symptoms

The patient may present with:
Pain
Deformity if there is a bony injury.
External signs of trauma such as bruising or laceration.
Urinary problems of haematuria, dysuria or retention.
It is important to observe for blood in the urethra as this usually indicates a ruptured urethra. This should be **notified** immediately.

If the patient with pelvic injuries has retention and a very distended bladder do **not** catheterize until the doctor has ensured that there is no uretheral damage. If there is damage, to remove the urine from the bladder the doctor will insert a catheter through the abdominal wall into the bladder, a suprapubic catheter. It is important to note in the female patient that a urethral tear may also be associated with a vaginal tear.

Patient Care

1 The importance of regular, accurate observations every 15 minutes can never be over emphasized. The patient with pelvic injuries can lose a considerable amount of blood from an internal haemorrhage. Be alert for the signs and symptoms of shock and prepare for the appropriate treatment.
2 Observe the type and severity of pain.
3 The moving of this patient must be carried out skillfully to prevent further damage from the fractured bones. Ambulance personnel are fully trained in the movement of these patients and will most probably have transferred the patient in a recumbent or semirecumbent position on a stretcher known as a scoop stretcher. This stretcher divides into 2 parts which allows it to be placed under the patient or removed from the patient with very little movement of the patient. Ensure that when the ambulance personnel bring the patient to the department that, when possible, the patient is placed on a trolley suitable for X-rays. This will mean that the patient does not have to be moved again.
4 In cases of suspected fractures of the pelvis or hips it is important to have two nurses present to undress the patient to allow for equal movement of the patient. Clothes should be removed with the patient in a recumbent or semirecumbent position without the patient moving from side to side and

without creating a force on the pelvic girdle. It may be necessary to cut off tight trousers.

5   Prepare an intravenous infusion. Fluid loss will need to be replaced so, depending on the severity of the patient's condition, plasma or cross-matched blood may be required.

6   If the patient wishes to pass urine the doctor should be notified as it is important to ensure first that there is no rupture to the bladder, otherwise, when the patient attempts to void, the urine will be expelled into the peritoneal cavity resulting in peritonitis.

The urine must be observed for haematuria. It must also be observed as to whether the patient has dysuria as this might indicate injury to the urethra or nerve damage. Lower abdominal injury may have affected the nerves of the sacral plexus. The sacral plexus is formed by the nerves which leave the spinal cord from the lumbar and sacral region. The nerves pass through the pelvic cavity and form the sciatic and other nerves of the leg. Injury to these nerves may result in retention of urine or the patient may complain of numbness in the legs.

If the patient is unable to pass urine but does not have a distended bladder this could indicate a possible ruptured bladder. In this case urine will leak into the pelvic cavity and the patient will present with problems of peritonitis.

7   In the case of a female patient it is important to move the patient as little as possible should she wish to urinate so instead of a bedpan the nurse may use a slipper pan (if the department has one) or a kidney dish placed in the appropriate position. Particular care must be taken on moving the legs; they must be moved slowly and together and as little as possible when placing the pan in position. Two nurses are required to assist the patient.

8   If the patient has nausea or vomiting observations should be made on the stomach contents. If there is haematemesis this **must** be reported immediately.

The stomach contents may consist of:
 Fresh blood indicating bleeding from the stomach.
 Altered blood — looks like coffee grounds and has remained in the stomach or duodenum long enough to undergo changes due to digestive processes.

Vomiting may require the passing of a nasogastric tube which must be on free drainage or aspirated at hourly intervals. Bleeding from further along the digestive tract may pass through the tract and be eliminated as melaena.

Treatment

Treatment in the form of surgical intervention will depend on the severity of the patient's condition and its necessity. Operations will be performed for ruptured ureters, bladder, urethra and to control severe internal haemorrhage. Surgery may also be necessary for the treatment of fractures, although fractures of the pelvis usually heal without surgical intervention.

FRACTURES

A fracture is an injury to the bone involving a break in the continuity of the bone. Normal bone is dense, strong tissue and to allow a break to occur usually requires force. The force which breaks the bone can vary in strength, location and direction of the blow resulting in different injuries.

Types of Fractures

A **simple** (closed) fracture is a single break in the bone with no communication to an external wound (Figure 55a).
A **compound** (open) fracture is a single break in the bone which has created a wound in the skin which directly communicates with the fracture (Figure 55c).
A **complicated** fracture is a single break in the bone where the broken ends of the bone do not communicate with a skin wound but injure other organs, e.g., lungs, nerves or arteries.
A **comminuted** fracture is when the bone is splintered into several pieces (Figure 56b).
A **greenstick** fracture occurs in children before the bone has completely ossified. The bone does not break in two but bends and cracks.

Recognizing a Fracture

To recognize a fracture there may be:
History of a fall or injury.
Localized pain. The patient can generally point to the actual area where the bone is injured because of the pain.
Swelling. The immediate area may become swollen. This may be due to internal haemorrhage or the trauma of tissue damage.

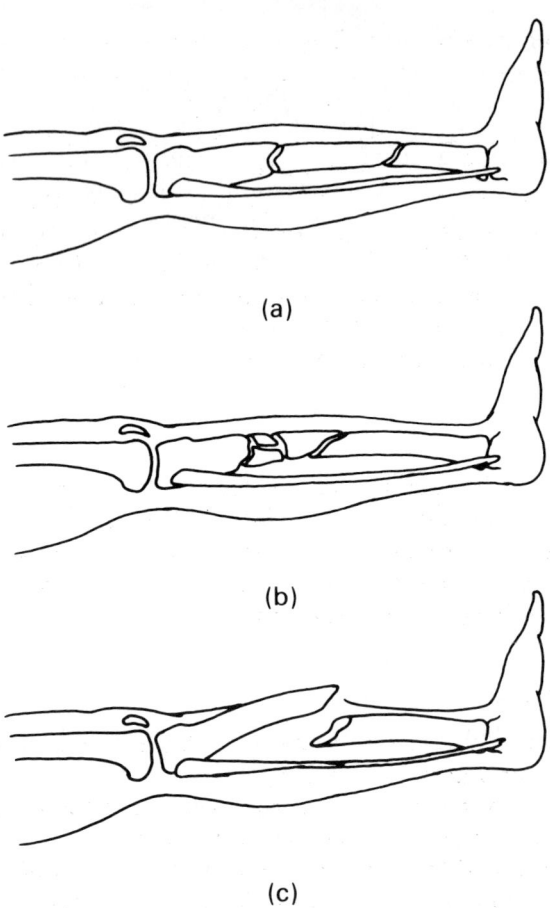

Figure 56 Types of fractures: simple (a); comminuted (b); compound (c).

Deformity. Deformity may be due to the muscles which are attached to the bones. Muscles usually work in pairs, while one muscle contracts the other relaxes allowing movement. The bone is the stable object the muscles pull against. Once the bone is fractured the muscles contract because they have nothing to pull against. This alters the position of the fractured area. For example, if a patient has fractured the neck of the femur then muscle contraction forces the leg to turn outwards (*abduction*). This results in the affected foot pointing sideways. It is also due to the muscle contraction that a fracture, which has occurred on a limb, can be recognized, because of the shortening of the limb.

Shortening of the limb. The fractured bone ends are pulled closer together (*impacted*) or pulled out of alignment by the contracted muscle and the result is a shorter limb.

Loss of normal function. As the muscles are unable to function correctly movement will be restricted and function limited. Pain also prevents the patient from moving the limb. If a nerve has been damaged by the fracture, in the case of a complicated fracture, then movement is altered and the patient may also complain of a disturbance in nerve sensations such as 'pins and needles' or numbness.

To confirm a fracture an X-ray will be taken.

Treatment

Treatment of fractures is often summarized under the following headings: resuscitation, reduction, restriction (immobilization), restoration and rehabilitation. Restoration involves restoring the patient to health through treatment, and rehabilitation involves prolonged physiotherapy.

Resuscitation

Resuscitation may be necessary as traumatic injuries often involve several areas of the body:

A patient may not have a fracture alone and the other injury may change the vital functions of the body.

Complications of fractures may affect other parts of the body, e.g. sternum or heart, often leading to a life-threatening situation.

Damage to bone can result in blood loss causing severe hypovolaemia and leaving the patient in a condition of shock. Blood loss from various fractures:

    Radius and ulna   250 ml
    Humerus   250–800 ml
    Pelvis   0.5–1 litre
    Femur   1–1.5 litres
    Tibia and fibula   250–750 ml

Assessment

Accurate assessment of the patient is essential to ascertain the necessity and immediacy of treatment:

1 Resuscitate
2 Treat the hypovolaemic condition
3 Prevent further damage — immobilization

Immobilization

A patient who enters the accident and emergency department with a suspected fracture must have the fracture immobilized. This is usually the responsibility of the nurse before the doctor sees the patient. The following fractures are best immobilized on admission by the following methods:

Clavicle. For a fractured clavicle — application of a sling. Clothing must be removed to allow the doctor a clear view of the affected site for examination. If the patient has loose fitting clothing then this does not necessarily need to be removed, especially if the patient is in severe pain.

Wrist. For a fractured wrist or Colles's fracture — application of a sling.

Ribs. For fractured ribs — if there is any skin injury this must be cleaned aseptically and covered with an air-tight dressing. Then application of a 15 cm crepe bandage around the chest against the skin.

Spine or Pelvis. For a fractured spine or pelvis — ensure that the patient is lying on a firm trolley with legs straight in a recumbent position (flat with one pillow behind the head). Remember if patient is having breathing difficulties this might be the most awkward position so allow a slight elevation of the trolley head. If the spine is injured in the region of the neck (cervical) then the patient should have sand bags placed on either side of the head to prevent any movement. Alternatively, if the patient needs to be more upright a correctly fitting cervical collar may be applied. To fit correctly the collar must completely prevent the patient's head from turning.

Femur. For a fractured femur — a full leg length back board or an air splint is required. Clothing will need to be removed from the affected leg for examination before the support is applied. If the patient has been brought to the hospital by ambulance the ambulance personnel will have already applied a splint. However, this will have to be removed for the clothing to be taken off. While the splint and clothing are being removed someone **must** maintain the position of the affected leg *and* prevent the muscles from contracting and causing further damage to the broken bone ends. The removal of clothing from a fractured leg therefore needs 3 people:

> One to hold the leg in extension by standing at the patient's feet, grasping the ankle with both hands and pulling gently away from the patient.
>
> Two to remove the clothing from the patient thus preventing the patient from having to turn.

It may be necessary to cut the clothing off the affected leg. Special care is needed in removing the boots worn by motor-cyclists who are often the victims of a fractured femoral shaft. The leg must be held as immobile as possible while the boot is removed. The nurse or ambulance personnel holding the leg will then need to hold the leg from the knee if a fractured femur is suspected or hold the ankle as the boot is removed if a fractured tibia and/or fibia are suspected. Once the clothing is removed then the splint must be applied. Only when the splint is applied should the leg be allowed to rest down without needing to be held.

Tibia and Fibula. For a fractured tibia or fibula — a back slab may be used. This is a board on which the leg rests. The leg may be held in position on the board by a bandage. Another method to secure the fracture is with an inflatable full leg splint. This is a clear double plastic bag shaped to fit over the leg secured with a zip-fastener or Velcro and can be inflated with air to hold it securely around the leg. The injured leg can be secured to the good leg to prevent unnecessary movement of the broken bone ends. The legs are secured together by bandages tied about the knees and around the ankles so that both legs move together from the joints and the fracture remains stable.

Ankle. For a fractured ankle or Pott's fracture — an inflatable boot is used. This is a shorter version of the full leg splint and measures from the patient's foot to below the knee.

For fractures of the tibia, fibula and ankle, care must be taken in removing footwear.

Rest of the fractured bone is essential to prevent further

damage and lessen the risk of fat embolus in shaft fractures. Restriction (immobilization) is the first care the fracture or suspected fracture must receive. Secondly if the fracture is compound, that is, if the fractured ends of the bones have a direct communication with a skin wound, the wound must be covered with an aseptic dressing. At this stage the wound should be **covered** and not cleaned as this will be done during surgery. Cleaning or attempting to clean the wound at this stage may cause additional injury to the fractured bone.

Reduction

Reduction is carried out following X-ray when a fracture is

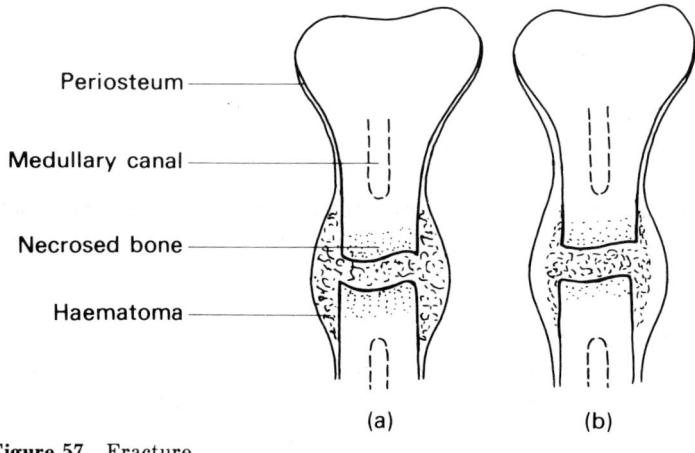

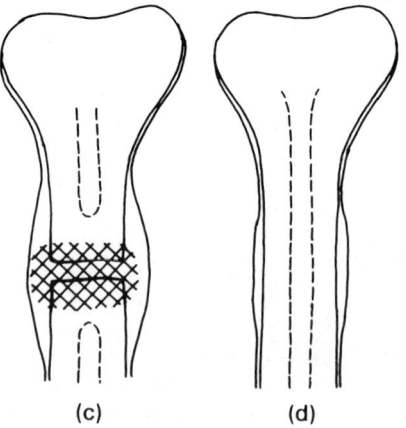

Figure 57 Fracture healing of a long bone: haematoma formation caused by blood from torn blood vessels (a); resolution of the haematoma and commencement of action by osteoclasts clearing away the necrosed bone (b); formation of a callus which occurs within 5 to 6 days (c); remodelling of the bone, by action of the osteoclasts which clear away excess bone material and osteoblasts which form new bone (d).

confirmed and located. Reduction means that the fractured ends of the bone are moved into alignment to allow healing to occur (Figure 57). Several methods of reduction may be used; the method depends on the type of fracture. The first decision is whether the fracture is simple (closed) or compound (open).

If the fracture is compound the patient is at risk to bacterial infection of the bone. To attempt to prevent this complication the fracture is treated in the sterile environment of the theatre, so a patient with a compound fracture must be prepared for a general anaesthetic (see p.73).

Sedation

Reduction is carried out in combination with one of the following forms of sedation.
1   Local anaesthetic
2   Intravenous Valium
3   General anaesthetic
4   Administration of entonox.

The choice of method is the decision of the doctor based on:
The age of the patient — children often require a general anaesthetic to allow bones to be repositioned.
The difficulty of realigning the fracture — the amount of muscle relaxation required.
The general physical condition of the patient. It is not advisable to subject patients with chronic lung or heart conditions to a general anaesthetic.
The time of the patient's last meal. If the patient has had a large meal within the last 4 - 6 hours a general anaesthetic would be inadvisable. The doctor will then decide whether to perform the reduction by local anaesthetic or to allow the patient to wait 4 - 6 hours before the procedure is undertaken.

Local Anaesthetic

Equipment required for a local anaesthetic (Buer block)
   Local anaesthetic — bupivacaine (Marcain)
   Syringe, needle
   Sphygmomanometer cuff
   Protection for the patient
   Equipment for the application of plaster:

Stockinette
Plaster of Paris bandages
Orthoban or similar padding
Bucket with tepid water
Scissors

The anaesthetist and doctor are present and the patient is prepared by being positioned on a trolley with the injured arm exposed. The patient is then protected by a plastic sheet. A sphygmomanometer cuff is placed around the upper part of the affected arm. The cuff is inflated to above the level of the patient's systolic blood pressure (this is achieved when there is no radial pulse present). It is generally the responsibility of the nurse to ensure that the cuff remains inflated during the procedure. The local anaesthetic is injected intravenously by the anaesthetist. The inflated sphygmomanometer cuff prevents the anaesthetic travelling throughout the blood stream. Skin changes will occur in the arm from the effects of the anaesthetic and lack of blood supply. It will turn pink and then a mottled white. Remember that the patient is conscious throughout this procedure so must be reassured and given explanations.

Reduction. Reduction can be carried out once the local anaesthetic has taken effect; the patient will be able to tell when there is no sensation of pain. The doctor can then manipulate the bone ends of the radius into position. When the bone is in alignment it must be held in that position and allowed to rest. For this reason plaster of Paris is applied. The plaster of Paris is usually formed on the upper side of the arm as a back slab so that the hand rests on the plaster but is not completely encased in plaster. The plaster is held against the arm by a crepe bandage. The wrist is not completely encased in plaster due to the swelling caused by the trauma.

When the wrist is immobilized in the plaster, or after 20 minutes, the sphygmomanometer cuff may be released slowly. It is important not to release the cuff before the 20 minutes period as the anaesthetic will still be effective and will circulate in the blood stream resulting in general effects.

Intravenous Valium

The preparation of a patient to receive intravenous Valium or a general anaesthetic is similar in some respects.

1 It is important to remove any dentures.
2 The patient should have an identification bracelet.
3 The patient should be undressed from above the waist and put in a theatre gown.
4 The patient should not have had a heavy meal within the last 4 hours.
Generally, it is the elderly or patients with chronic lung disease who are unsuitable for general anaesthesia.

General Anaesthetic

Preparation for a general anaesthetic must include:
1 The signing of a consent form.
2 Keeping the patient nil by mouth for 4 to 6 hours prior to surgery.
3 Removing any prosthesis.
4 Identifying the patient by placing an identification bracelet on the patient's wrist.

Patient Care. After the administration of intravenous Valium or a general anaesthetic, the after care of the patient involves:
1 Observations of airway, breathing and pulse.
2 Keeping the patient in the department until fully conscious.
3 Ensuring that there is someone to accompany the patient home.

Entonox

Entonox is a pain-relieving gas which is increasing in use in the accident and emergency department; it is a 50/50 mixture of oxygen and nitrous oxide. It may be used directly for pain relief especially in first aid or it may be used to relieve pain which will be experienced during such procedures as suturing or manipulation of fractures. It is commonly associated with childbirth.
   The advantage is that the patient does **not** loose consciousness and so is able to co-operate with the procedure.

Administration. With the administration of Entonox:
1 Ensure that the patient is sitting or lying down.
2 Instruct the patient to lift the mask to his or her face and place it securely over the nose and mouth. Ensure that the cylinder is switched on and then instruct the patient to breath

normally; within 20 seconds the patient should feel the effects.
3 It is important to inform the patient that there may be a sensation of dizziness and that this is normal. This is the reason why the patient must be in the position of sitting or lying.
4 Entonox is self-administered by breathing in via the mask. As soon as the patient feels relief it may be discontinued. The effects of the Entonox diminish as soon as atmospheric air is inhaled. If the patient requires further pain relief then breathing via the mast must be recommenced.

Entonox is extremely safe to use and does not interfere with other drugs, however it is an analgesic and must be administered with trained personnel in attendance.

Common Fracture Sites

Clavicle

The clavicle is a long, slender bone which forms part of the shoulder girdle. It articulates at one end with the scapula and at the other with the sternum. The clavicle is often injured when a person in falling extends an arm to 'break' the fall and thereby falls on the outstretched arm.

Signs and Symptoms. The signs and symptoms of a fractured clavicle are:
1 The patient will complain of pain in the region of the clavicle. Pain will increase on movement of the arm on the affected side. Movement of the arm will aggravate the fracture site and must be discouraged and the arm immobilized (see p.214).
2 Due to the pain the patient often appears pale and complains of faintness. Sitting or lying the patient down and supporting the affected arm alleviates the pain and also increases the blood supply to the brain thereby curing the feeling of faintness.

Treatment. The aim of treatment is to immobilize and hold the fractured clavicle in position. Immobilization can be achieved by the use of a sling or the application of a figure of eight bandage. Clothing, if not already removed, must be removed from above the waist. It is less distressful to the patient to remove clothing from the unaffected arm first, then the head and then slowly from the affected arm. Keep the patient in a warm environment if possible.

For a figure-of-eight bandage the following is required:
  2 gamgee pads
  1 roll of domette

To apply:
1 Sit the patient on a stool. This allows access to the back of the patient.
2 When possible, sit the patient in front of a mirror. Standing behind the patient you will be unable to observe the patient's face for pain or feelings of faintness. With the patient in front of a mirror, you can both be seen.
3 Standing behind, ask the patient to position the shoulders as far back as possible. This position is best achieved by asking the patient to place both hands on the hips, and pushing the elbows backwards.
4 Place a gamgee pad under each arm pit.
5 Start the figure-of-eight bandage on the unaffected side taking the domette down under the axilla then up and over the shoulder, (Figure 58a) and up over the affected shoulder and down under the axilla.
6 The bandage should be applied firmly with tension applied to position the shoulders back (Figure 58b).
7 On the third or fourth cross over at the back take the bandage up and behind the cross over (Figure 58c).
8 Wrap this domette round once and then fix with a safety pin (Figure 58d).
9 Check the radial pulse of the affected arm.
10 Make sure the patient does not complain of 'pins and needles' in the hands.
If the patient has any complaints the figure-of-eight must be reapplied. Absence of the radial pulse in the affected arm or a disturbance in nerve sensations to that arm means that the bandage is compressing the brachial artery and nerve in the region of the axilla.

Instructions for the patient:
1 The bandage is applied to keep the fracture in line. Therefore it needs to be kept in place and tightening as necessary.
2 Ordinary clothes can be worn over the bandage.
3 Return to accident and emergency or the fracture clinic to have the bandage reapplied in 2 to 3 days; or return to the fracture clinic for an appointment.

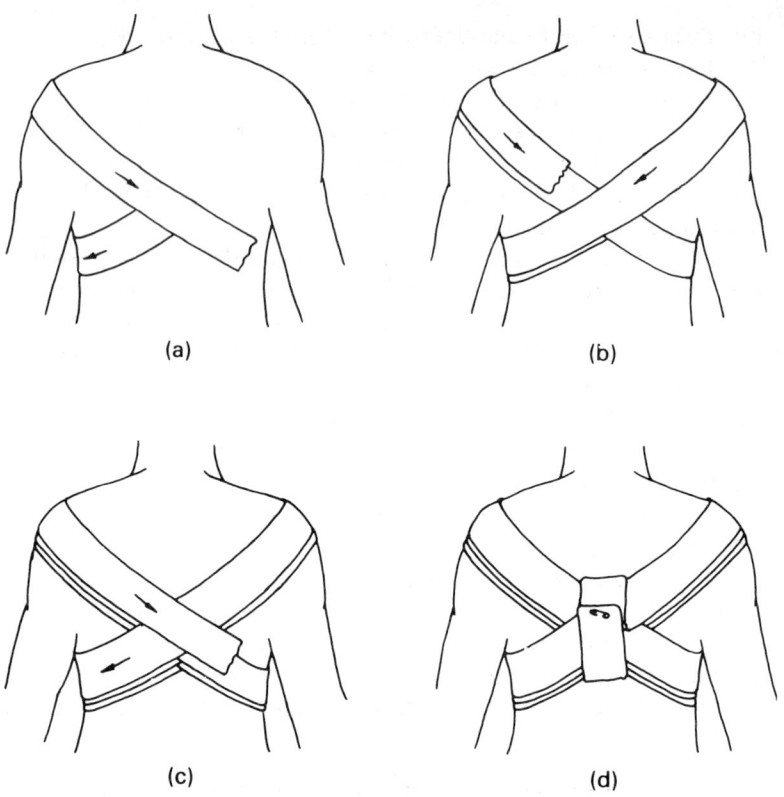

Figure 58 Application of a figure-of-eight bandage: the domette is placed on the unaffected shoulder first (a), and then applied around the affected shoulder (b). This procedure is followed three or four times (c), and the bandage secured with a safety pin (d).

Wrist

A common fracture to the wrist is a *Colles's fracture*. It is a fracture of the distal end of the radius and is frequently seen in the accident and emergency department especially when icy conditions prevail. The patient presents with a history of a fall on to the hand, and a typical 'dinner fork deformity'. Another bone of the wrist which is commonly fractured is one of the eight carpals, the scaphoid. This bone directly articulates with the radius.

Signs and Symptoms. The signs and symptoms of a Colles's fracture are:
1 Localized pain

2   Deformity and swelling due to tissue injury
3   Immobility of fingers

Treatment. Treatment is reduction (see p.216) once the wrist is supported in a sling. Following this a slab is applied (see p.249). Some departments will have the patient's wrist X-rayed following reduction, while others require the patient to return the next day. The patient must know when and where.

Scaphoid Fracture

A scaphoid fracture may not show on the initial X-ray and the wrist may have been treated by being rested with a strapping bandage (see Chapter 4). The patient could then complain of continual problems with the wrist and follow-up X-rays at 7 and 21 days reveal the fracture by the line of calcification which appears across the scaphoid. The fracture may then be treated with a plaster of Paris cast.

Discharging a Patient. On discharge from the department the nurse must ensure that the patient will be able to manage:
1   Manage day to day living activities — if unable, arrange social service assistance.
2   Arrange transport to and from the hospital — it may be necessary to arrange ambulance transportation for the clinic appointments.

Ribs

The ribs form part of the thoracic cage. There are 12 pairs of ribs each one being an elongated flat bone. The ribs all articulate with the thoracic vertebrae of the spinal cord.
Anteriorly some ribs join with the sternum and these ribs are known as *true ribs*. The first 7 pairs of ribs are the true ribs.
The eighth, ninth and tenth are known as *false ribs* as they articulate with each other and not the sternum.
The eleventh and twelfth pairs of ribs are embedded in muscle and are known as *floating ribs*.

Signs and Symptoms
1   The patient will complain of pain especially on respiration and will be reluctant to take deep breaths or cough.

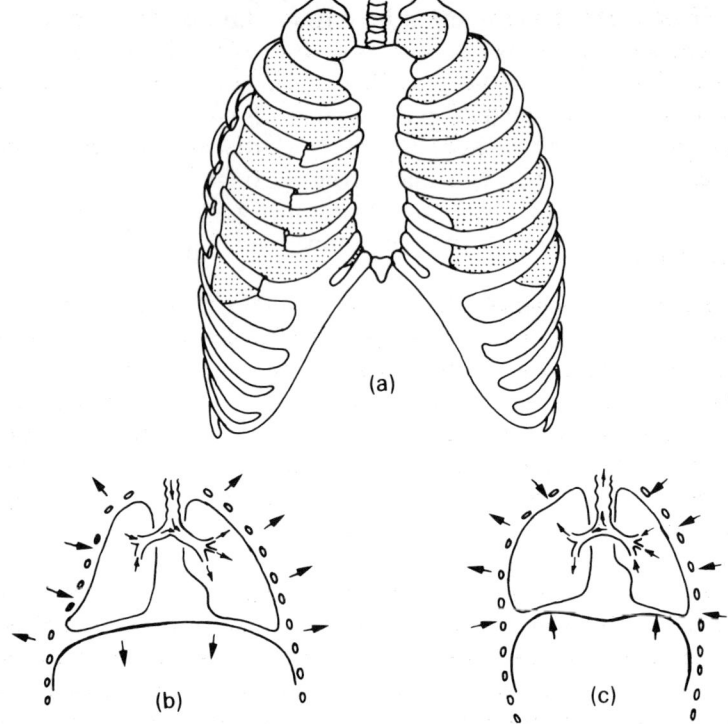

Figure 59 Flail chest occurs when there is more than one fracture on the same rib, or closely related ribs (a), results in an alteration of the respiratory mechanism; on inspiration (b), the area of the fractured ribs moves in apposition to normal chest movement *(arrows)*; on expiration (c), the area of he fractured ribs moves outwards in apposition to normal chest movement *(arrows)*.

2 Bruising may appear at the site of the injury.
3 The chest may move unequally. If more than one fracture has been sustained on the same rib or on several related ribs the patient will develop the condition of a flail chest (Figure 59).

Treatment
1 Rib fractures often unite without any intervention. However, support by firm bandaging prevents the patient from suffering too much discomfort.
2 Analgesia is usually required. The patient must be encouraged to take deep breaths and to cough to keep the chest clear of infection but many will be reluctant to do this if it is painful.

3 If the rib fracture or the chest trauma has caused a pneumothorax (allowed air into the pleural space) or a haemothorax (caused bleeding within the pleural space) then this must be treated (see p.201).
The patient will require hospital admission for rest and observation.

Flail Chest

The nurse will observe a flail chest by seeing that on inspiration, when the ribs should move up and out, the part of the ribs fractured will move in the opposite direction, moving inwards. This is because the fractured segment of rib or ribs is not controlled by the remainder of the thoracic cavity and therefore is unable to move with it. The result is that the fractured segment on inspiration moves inwards and compresses the lung, and moves outwards on expiration.

Treatment. The treatment for this is, as for any fracture, to immobilize the fracture. A firm crepe bandage around the chest will support the area. Also the patient can be turned on to the effected side again as a support. This support is particularly important during the time of expiration because as the rib cage moves down and in to its original position the flail (fracture) segment moves outwards in the opposite direction.

SPINAL INJURIES

Various injuries can occur to the spinal column and the related tissues. The spinal column forms part of the axial skeleton and consists of 33 bones or vertebrae. The bones are named and numbered according to their location (Table 8). The vertebrae

Table 8 The bones of the spinal column.

Location	Number of vertebrae
Cervical (neck region)	7
Thoracic (dorsal region)	12
Lumbar	5
Sacral	5
Coccyx	4

are separated from each other by intervertebral discs. These discs are flexible, elastic sections of cartilage which cushion the vertebra and allow some movement of the spine.

Types of Injury

Various injuries can occur to the spinal column:

Muscular. Muscular injuries occur especially in the cervial region (*torticollis*). This is not always related to injury but causes the patient pain. The muscles are severely contracted and the head (in torticollis) is pulled over to one side due to muscle contraction.

Disc Lesion. Disc lesions tend to occur in the cervical and lumbar region. They can be due to injuries such as falling or often, in the case of a lumbar disc lesion, from bending over or lifting incorrectly. Whatever the reason the disc has moved from its normal position *(prolapse)*.

Fracture of the Vertebra. Sudden compression on the spinal cord, such as occurs when falling heavily while upright, may result in a fracture of the vertebrae. Fractures can occur in other parts of the vertebrae apart from the body and may be associated with dislocation, due to rupture of the supporting ligaments. A cause of this injury is the whip lash injury to the neck of a passenger when a car stops suddenly. These injuries can all result in damage to the spinal cord and its nerves.

Spinal Cord

The spinal cord is contained within the spinal column along with the meninges, the cerebrospinal fluid and blood vessels. The spinal cord consists of nerve fibres which extend from the foramen magnum at the base of the skull to the lower end of the first lumbar vertebra. Extending from the spinal cord are 31 pairs of spinal nerves. Each pair corresponds with a vertebra and supplies a different part of the body. The spinal nerves are responsible for peripheral nerve response via the reflex arc which produce reflex actions (Figure 60).

Damage to the spinal cord can alter the central nervous system control and the reflex action of the spinal nerves. The

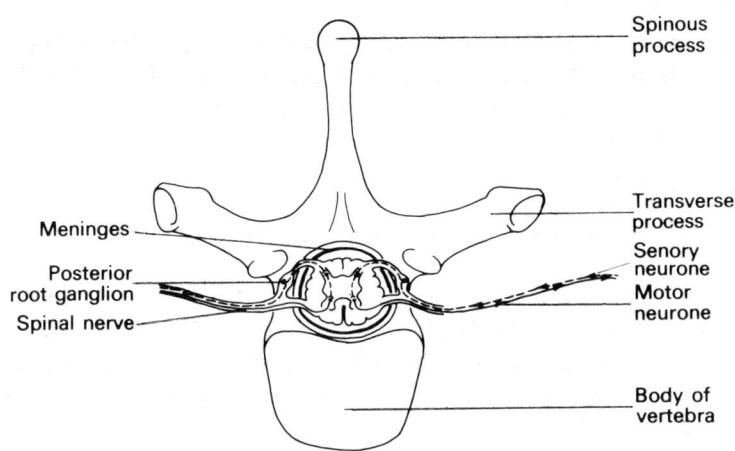

Figure 60 Cross-section of the spinal cord, showing the pathway of the nerve impulses (arrows) which comprise of the sensory neurone (hatched line) and the motor neurone (solid line) and are related to reflex actions.

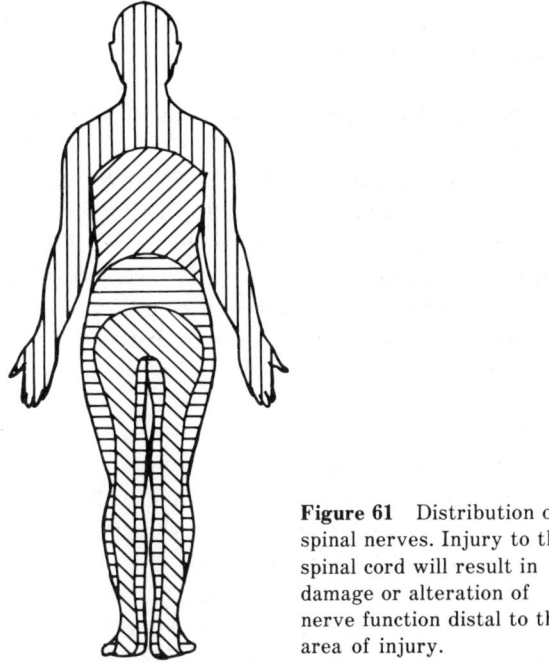

Figure 61 Distribution of spinal nerves. Injury to the spinal cord will result in damage or alteration of nerve function distal to the area of injury.

area of the body affected depends on the area of the spinal cord and the spinal nerves which are injured (Figure 61).

If the spinal cord is affected in the cervical or thoracic region, the patient's respiratory function may be disturbed.

Damage in the lumbar region will result in alteration of sensation to the legs but may also produce incontinence in the patient due to the alteration of the nerve function to the bladder and bowel spincters.

Patient Care

1 Assess the priorities. All spinal injuries are treated as unstable until they are proved otherwise.

2 **Do not** move the patient until the injuries are assessed and appropriate measures are taken in movement. This means the affected limbs must be immobilized and the spinal column supported. A patient with spinal injuries **must** be placed in a recumbent position with arms and legs straight and head supported between two sand bags to prevent movement. If it is necessary to maintain the patient's airway then this must be done by using a Guedel airway as further damage can result from turning the patient's head onto the side or from moving the patient to a semiprone position.

To remove the patient's clothing 2 or more nurses will be needed. The patient can be undressed from the upper part of the body by both the patient's arms being lifted above the head and the clothing pulled upwards from the patient's body, finally being released from the arms. Garments can be removed from the lower part of the body by slight elevation of the buttocks and gentle even movement from both sides.

3 If the injury has resulted in a disturbance of nerve sensation, be particularly aware of pressure areas. The patient will require correct handling and positioning of the affected area and will require relief of pressure areas at least every 2 hours. If the patient remains in the department for over 2 hours, the nurse will need to know the extent of the injury and how much movement of the patient is advised so that action can be taken to prevent pressure areas becoming pressure sores. When the patient is admitted to the ward it is necessary to tell the ward staff of the altered sensations so that necessary aids for pressure relief may be put into the bed before the patient is transferred from the trolley.

4 If the patient is complaining of pain the doctor must be informed so that it can be decided whether the patient may have an analgesic.

Treatment

For a spinal injury, treatment may involve the application of traction. The types of traction depend on the area of injury. The aim of traction in this case is to keep the vertebrae in position and aligned to prevent pressure on the spinal cord or nerves.

    Skeletal skull traction — for cervical injuries with the head of the bed elevated.
    Lumbar/Sacral traction — skin traction to legs with foot of the bed elevated.

Traction is generally applied when the patient is transferred to the ward.

Psychological Care

Spinal injuries are generally painful and disabling. Patients will worry about whether they will be able to straighten up again, move or even walk again. In the initial stages of the injury the actual effects are often difficult to predict so that patients can not always be given a definite answer. However, explanations of treatment and alleviation of pain will help relieve the patient's anxiety.

PELVIC INJURIES

Pelvic injuries are generally caused by violent force such as a road traffic accident. The pelvic girdle consists of 2 hip bones and the sacrum. The 2 hip bones join anteriorly at the symphysis pubis. The hip bones each consist of 3 bones: the ilium, the ischium and the pubis. These bones unite together at the acetabulum. The acetabulum is the cup-shaped socket into which the head of the femur fits.

Signs and Symptoms

The signs and symptoms are generally the same as those for a patient with lower abdominal injuries, and pelvic fractures often cause complications of internal injury.

Remember blood loss may be considerable; the patient may be in:
    Shock
    Considerable pain

Internal damage may result in a ruptured bladder, ureter, urethra, bowel or vagina. Any unnatural drainage into the pelvic cavity, such as urine, will lead to peritonitis. Therefore, moving and positioning the patient is especially important (see Chapter 2).

Patient Assessment

Assess the patient's condition:
1   Observe the patient every 15 minutes.
2   Urine tests — observe whether the patient has dysuria, haematuria, anuria or retention.
3   Report immediately if patient has bleeding per urethra or vagina as this may indicate a rupture.

Treatment

The patient will be admitted to the ward and may require surgery for the internal injury (see p.208) or skin traction to treat the fractured pelvis. Rarely do pelvic fractures require surgery but this may be necessary to bring the fracture into alignment.

INJURIES TO THE LIMBS

Upper Limbs

The upper limbs or arms consist of typical long bones. The humerus is the bone of the upper arm and the head of this bone fits into the glenoid cavity of the scapula of the shoulder joint. The radius and ulna are the bones of the forearm. Fractures can occur to the humerus, radius and ulna.

Signs and Symptoms

The characteristic signs and symptoms of a fractured arm include:
Pain. The patient will complain of localized pain.
Trauma. There will be a history of trauma. These fractures can present from a direct force or an indirect force which has twisted the bone and caused it to fracture.

Simple fractures of the humerus in children before the bones have completely ossified are unusual. The fracture will have required a violent force which cannot be produced by a child tripping over as the weight would not be sufficient. However, there may be a history of a fall from a height or an accident; or child abuse may be the cause (see Chapter 12). The distal end of the humerus is designed to form the hinge joint with the radius and ulna. The change in shape at the end of the humerus forms the condyles and the greater tuberosity for the joint. Just above the condyles are the median nerve and the brachial artery which are the nerve and blood supply to the lower arm. A fracture in this region (*supracondylar fracture*) can damage the artery and the nerve. Patients with a supracondylar fracture are admitted to hospital so that regular observations of the radial pulse may be recorded.

Treatment

Treatment of an arm fracture includes:
1 Immobilization with a sling except in the case of supracondylar fractures where flexion may cause further damage to the median nerve. For a supracondylar fracture support the patient's arm on a pillow but do not move the arm from the position the patient has it in on admission.
2 Reduction of the fracture by general anaesthetic within the department or on admission to hospital. If the fracture is not displaced the patient will not require reduction but will have a plaster of Paris applied to ensure that the fractured bone ends remain in position until the bone ends have formed a stable union.
3 Following reduction, restriction (rest) will be maintained by the application of a full plaster of Paris.

After Care

If the patient has been treated in the department and is discharged home ensure that complete instructions are given as to the care of the plaster. The arm must be elevated in a sling or by using a collar and cuff sling (see Chapter 4). Do not use a collar and cuff sling if the patient has an injured wrist as this will aggravate the wrist injury.

Dislocation

A dislocation means the movement of a bone from its normal position of function. In the case of the shoulder it means that the head of the humerus has moved out of the glenoid cavity so that the ball and socket joint is no longer intact or able to facilitate movement. The injury occurs when someone falls heavily on his or her shoulder.

Signs and Symptoms

The patient complains of severe pain in the shoulder, an inability to move the arm and may be clutching the arm to prevent movement. The pain, as with a fractured clavicle, may make the patient feel nauseated and faint. The patient should sit with the arm supported in a sling or be placed on a trolley with arm resting on a pillow and across the chest. Clothing must be removed from the upper part of the body to facilitate the doctor's examination.

Treatment

The main treatment is reduction and this means moving the bone into its correct position. The procedure will be carried out by the doctor. To allow movement of the humerus back into position the patient will require some form of sedation. Entonox may be used, or an intravenous injection of Valium or a general anaesthetic. The patient must be prepared appropriately (see p.217).

After Care

It is important to make sure that the shoulder does not dislocate again so the arm must be held in adduction. The position can be obtained by the patient positioning the arm across the chest. The arm may be held in this position by a sling and further secured with a crepe bandage around the chest or by a netalast dressing. As the patient must retain this position for approximately 2 - 3 weeks the sling and bandage are applied under the clothing. The patient will return for a check-up in 2 - 3 weeks and to the physiotherapy department for arm exercises.

Following reduction the pain subsides.

The patient must be encouraged to exercise the fingers of the injured arm.

On Discharge

Ensure that the patient is able to get home and can manage once there.

INJURIES TO THE LOWER LIMBS

The lower limbs consist of the bone of the upper leg, that is, the femur, being the longest bone in the body and the bones of the lower leg, the tibia and fibula. The proximal end of the femur forms the head of the femur which is designed to fit into the acetabulum formed by the pelvic bones. This is a synovial joint or ball and socket joint and allows movement of the lower limbs and trunk. The head of the femur narrows as it joins the main shaft of the femur forming the neck of the femur. It is this point of the femur which is most commonly fractured.

Dislocation of the Hip

With dislocation of the hip, the head of the femur has moved out of the acetabulum (Figure 62). This may occur as a complication

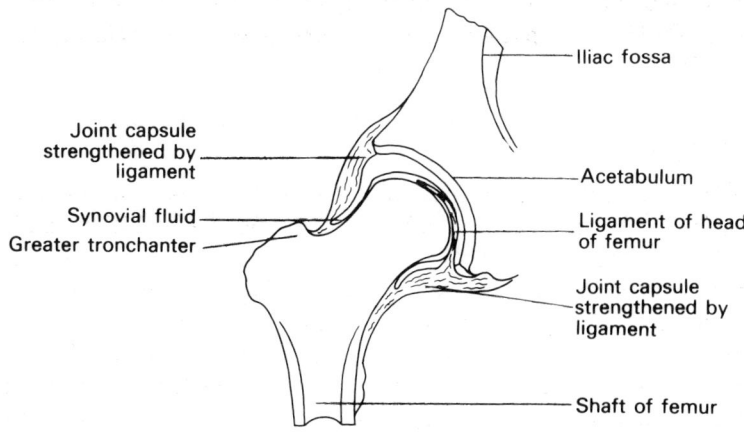

Figure 62 A synovial joint — the hip joint.

following the insertion of an artificial femoral head, such as a Monks prothesis. Following the surgical procedure the patient is nursed with the affected leg abducted to keep the prosthesis in the acetabulum.

Trauma also causes dislocation, generally as a result of a direct force against the knee with the patient in a sitting position, e.g., when driving a car. The direct force pushes the knee and femur backwards and forces the head of the femur out of the acetabulum.

Signs and Symptoms

With a dislocated hip there may be:
    A history of trauma
    Complaints from the patient of severe pain in the region of the hip.
    Disturbance in the movement of the limb
    Possibly damage to the nerve or blood supply to the limb.

Patient Care

1 Position the patient on a trolley in a semirecumbent position. Placing a pillow under the knee of the affected leg may help to alleviate the pain.
2 Undress the lower limbs of the patient with care. Remove clothing from the unaffected limb first.
3 Assess the patient for other injuries. Remember this injury is often caused by a road traffic accident.
4 Observe the limb for alteration in blood supply or nerve sensations.
5 Give analgesia if prescribed by the doctor.
6 Prepare the patient for a general anaesthetic or sedation by Valium to allow the bone to be replaced.

After Care

After care involves keeping the affected leg abducted to maintain the position of the head of the femur. The patient will be admitted to hospital for rest of the affected area and for observations.

Dislocation of the Patella

When the patella moves out of position it is said to be dislocated. The patella (knee cap) is a bone within a tendon and is round, flat and articulates with the femur. Dislocation of the patella can occur during sporting activity and may reoccur in the same patient.

Signs and Symptoms

With dislocation of the patella there may be:
Pain around the knee
Inability to straighten the leg. The patient may tend to hop clutching the leg.

Treatment

1 Place the patient on a trolley and gently straighten the leg.
2 Remove lower clothing.
3 On the doctor's examination the patella can usually be manipulated into position and the patient rarely requires an anaesthetic.

After Care

To prevent further injury, after care involves the knee being supported by a Robert Jones bandage (see p. 91).
The patient is generally discharged home and advised not to put any weight on the leg for 3 to 4 days.
Make sure that the patient is provided with crutches and can manage with them (see p. 95).

Fractured Femoral Neck

A fractured femoral neck is a common injury seen in an accident and emergency department. It is generally an injury which occurs to the elderly. For this reason the overall assessment must include the patient's general condition.

An elderly patient may have fallen initially as the result of health problems such as dizziness or poor eyesight and once fallen may have been unable to get up again and, consequently have additional problems of hypothermia due to immobility or may have been incontinent.

Signs and Symptoms

With a fractured femoral neck there may be:
  A history of trauma.
  Pain localized in the limp.
  Shortening of the affected limb due to muscle contraction.
  External rotation of the limb.
  Difficulty in weight bearing on the affected limb or in movement.
A patient has been known to walk into the accident and emergency department with a fractured femoral neck complaining only of a slight pain in the hip.

Patient Care

1 Position the patient on a secure trolley and undress the patient carefully making sure that the lower limbs are always in alignment.
2 Observe for any other signs of injury by assessing the patient.
3 Reassure and explain to the patient. Remember elderly patient may have difficulty in seeing or hearing and may be confused in a strange environment.
4 Protect the patient from further injury. If the patient is confused and restless make sure someone, a nurse, relative or friend, is with the patient at all times, to prevent another fall. Always have the sides of the trolley elevated, this prevents the patient from falling off the trolley and allows a feeling of security if the patient has something to hold on to.
5 Administer analgesia when prescribed.
6 If a bedpan is required allow the patient privacy and time. Always ensure that there are two nurses to put the patient onto the bed pan. Remember to test the urine and to record the result, trauma may have affected the bladder or urethra.

Treatment

Treatment will inovlve admission to hospital and an operation. Surgery may not be immediate but performed in several days time.
Make sure that the next of kin is informed.

The immediate care involves reduction and rest. This is achieved by the application of skin traction to the affected leg. This is generally applied when the patient is transferred to the ward.

Fractured Femoral Shaft

Fracture of the femoral shaft is caused by a violent force and may result in a blood loss of 1 to 1.5 litres.

Signs and Symptoms

Signs and symptoms of a fractured femoral shaft may include:
Extreme pain localized to the site of the fracture.
Disturbance in movement.
Shortening of the affected leg.
External rotation due to muscle contraction.
Localized swelling due to tissue traum and internal haemorrhage.

Patient Care

1 Position the patient on a firm trolley in a semirecumbent position.
2 Undress the patient ensuring that the affected leg is held immobile (see p.214).
3 Assess patient, remember internal haemorrhage may present a patient in the condition of shock and there may also be other injuries.
4 Prepare an intravenous infusion for the doctor to commence, to treat the condition of shock.
5 Give analgesia if ordered.
6 Following the doctor's examination, traction is applied with the aid of a Thomas' splint. This may be applied in the accident and emergency department.

Fixed Traction. For the application of skin traction, the leg must be held to maintain the fracture position while traction is applied (Figure 63a). The traction will be held in place by crepe bandages (Figure 63b). The Thomas' splint is applied to allow fixed traction. The splint consists of a ring attached to parallel longitudinal bars. The ring goes around the top of the leg and must be measured to ensure that the splint fits correctly. The circumference of the leg is measured at the groin and the length of the leg is taken from the top of the leg to the heel of the foot

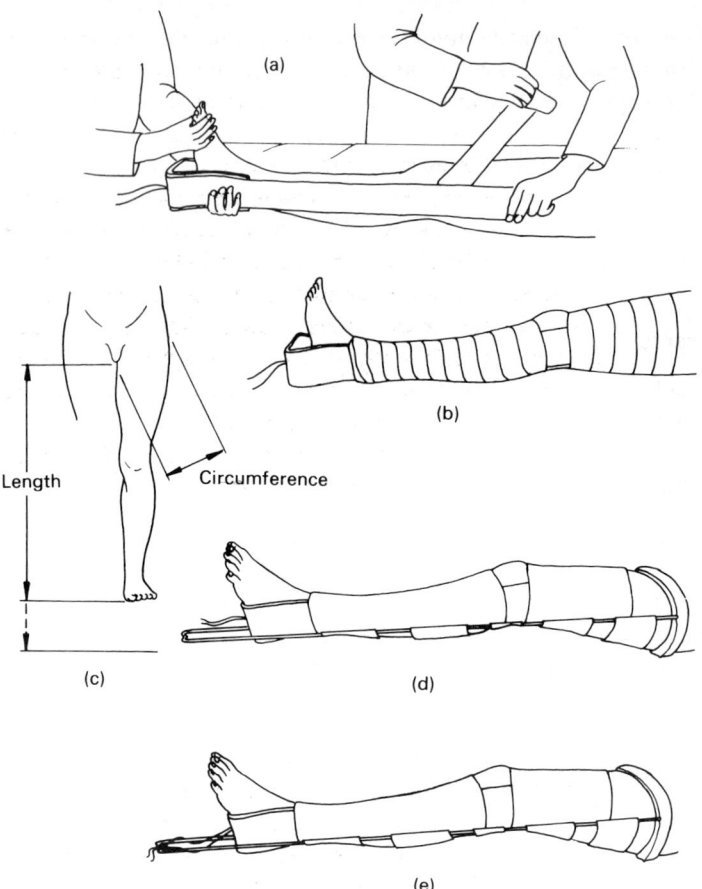

Figure 63 Application of skin traction: leg must be held to maintain fracture position (a); traction is secured by crepe bandages (b). The application of a Thomas' splint: splint must be measured for the patient (c); leg is positioned in the Thomas' splint (d); skin traction is tied securely to the Thomas' splint (e).

plus 20–30 cm (Figure 63c). The leg is positioned resting on domette in the Thomas' splint (Figure 63d). The skin traction is then tied securely to the splint ensuring traction on the leg (Figure 63e).

Treatment

For treatment the patient will require admission to hospital. If the fractured bone ends are not aligned by traction they will rquire open surgery. this may involve the insertion of a pin throughout the shaft of the femur, e.g., Kuntscher nail, or the insertion of a plate over the fracture lines which is held in place with screws. If the fracture shaft of femur produced bone ends which were in communication with a skin wound, a compound fracture, the patient would require surgery for aseptic toileting and realignment of fracture and admission to hospital.

The nurse should place a sterile dressing over the patient's communicating skin wound on the patient's admission to the department.

Fracture of Tibia and Fibula

Fractures of the tibia or the fibula or both are often the result of sporting or motor-bicycle injuries. The tibia is the larger weight-bearing bone of the lower leg. The fibula lies parallel and slightly behind the tibia. Observe as to whether these injuries have formed compound fractures and treat accordingly.

Signs and Symptoms

The signs and symptoms of a fractured tibia or fibula, as with all other fractures include:
    Localized pain
    Difficulty in movement
    Deformity of affected limb

Patient Care

1 Remove clothing from area with care. Immobilize once clothing is removed. This is best obtained by using a leg-length air splint. Ensure that an aseptic dressing is placed over the wound of a compound fracture before an air splint is applied.
2 Assess the patient for any other trauma.
3 Observe the affected leg for signs of swelling and circulatory deficiency.
4 Does the patient have the sensation of 'pins and needles' in the affected leg or is the leg sensitive to touch indicating possible nerve damage.
5 Prepare the patient for surgery and admission if it is a compound fracture.
6 Depending on the severity of the fracture, whether it is simple, complicated or comminuted, prepare the patient for a general anaesthetic.

Treatment

A simple fracture may be treated in the department and reduced under a general anaesthetic and the patient discharged home with a full leg plaster. Other fractures, if not easily reduced, will necessitate the admission of the patient to hospital.

Pott's Fracture

Fractures of the lower end of the tibia and fibula at the ankle are known as a Pott's fracture. These fractures cause pain, swelling and an inability to bear one's own weight. The patient is often treated in the department, having a reduction under a general anaesthetic or sedation by Valium. The patient is discharged home with a knee-length plaster with instructions not to bear weight on the injured limb for 48 hours, which means that the patient requires crutches and also information on how to look after the plaster. The patient must be advised when and where to return.

Complications

Much of the nursing in the accident and emergency department, apart from treating the actual condition, is aimed at observing for and preventing complications. The first three possible complications should always be considered by the nurse during care of the patient:

Shock — due to hypovolaemia
Infection
Injury to nerves and blood vessels

Later complications can include:

Deformity — obvious on initial injury but on healing may still be present.
Stiffness of joints — due to immobility while fracture site was restricted.
Non-union — when reduction has not successfully brought the bone ends into alignment.
Muscle wastage — due to inactivity.
A deep vein thrombosis.

One other important complication of a fracture, particularly of a long bone, can develop within 48 hours of injury. That is, after a fracture, fat globules are released in the bloodstream (emboli) and cause complete obstructin to small blood vessels, especially in the lungs, brain and kidneys. The patient presents with symptoms according to the area affected. Prompt and effective immobilization will help to prevent this potentially fatal complication of fat emboli.

PLASTERING

Basic Principles of Making a Cast

Before padding or constructing a cast, it is imperative that the nurse ensures that there is an adequate supply of padding and Gypsona bandages in the various sizes required. All materials and instruments should be carefully laid out within easy reach; delay caused by inadequate preparation is the greatest cause of delamination and weakness in the cast.

Padding

The unpadded splint provides more efficient support than a padded plaster cast because it is close to the bone. However, in the following circumstances, padded casts are more suitable and safer:
- Where swelling is present or suspected, i.e., in almost every acute condition.
- When the limb is thin and the bones are very superficial.
- When wedging is contemplated.
- When electric plaster cutters are used for removal of the cast.

With the patient correctly positioned and the injured limb supported, orthopaedic padding of the required width is unrolled and firmly applied over the full area of the limb to be covered by the plaster.

Preparing Gypsona Bandages

Gypsona bandages should be prepared individually:
1 Unroll the first 10–15 cm to allow identification of the free end before soaking and hold the bandage lightly in one hand, with the little finger supporting one end of the plastic core.
2 Immerse the bandage at an angle of 45° in a standard 9-litre bucket of cool water (23–35°C) and soak until bubbling ceases

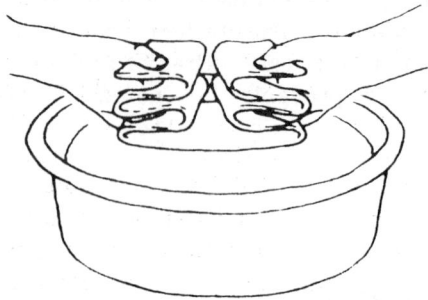

Figure 64 After soaking the bandage, remove the bandage from the water and gently squeeze the ends of the roll to expel excess water.

(approximately 5 seconds). Cooler water extends the setting time.

3 Withdraw the bandage, and using both hands, gently squeeze the ends of the roll simultaneously to expel excess water (Figure 64). Do **not** wring. This ensures that the plaster cream remains within the bandage and is not expelled from the ends of the rolls by uneven squeezing.

Points to Remember

Four important points to remember:

1 Always change the water after it has been used for soaking 6-8 bandages since it will have become supersaturated with calcium sulphate and will impair effective soaking for subsequent bandages.

2 Rinse hands frequently in order to keep them free from hard plaster particles.

3 Do not soak more than 1 bandage at a time. The reason for this is that setting commences immediately the bandage is in contact with water, and while 1 bandage is being applied, those left soaking will also have started to set, thereby reducing the time available for preparing the cast.

4 Protect unused bandages from accidental splashing by keeping them well away from water at all times.

Preparing the Cast

Having applied the padding, the nurse rolls the bandage evenly round the limb, without undue tension, which could result in constriction if the limb is swollen, and without wrinkling, which could result in pressure sores. To ensure that the bandage lies smoothly and that it follows the contours of the limb, pleats should be made where necessary at the upper or lower edges of the bandages. However, the edge of a bandage should never coincide with a crease in the skin, since this could result in pressure sores. As each bandage is applied, it should be constantly moulded and smoothed with the wet palms. This ensures that the layers will be bonded into an homogeneous mass and that the cast will be strong and well-fitting. If this is not carried out, delamination may occur, resulting in a weakened cast. It is essential that the moulding of each bandage is completed while the plaster is still workable, otherwise crystallization of the plaster may be disturbed, resulting in a weakened cast. As the plaster sets, heat is generated and the patient should be assured that this is normal.

During the moulding, care must be taken to ensure that only the palms of the hands are used and that the fingers do not cause indentations which could lead to pressure sores. If during application of the bandage the threads unravel, they should be cut to prevent any possibility of constriction.

To ensure that a free range of movements is possible at the joints not immobilized, the edges of the wet cast should be trimmed and smoothed. If stockinette padding is used, this should be turned back over the edge of the plaster and kept neatly in place by strips of bandage. Just before the plaster finally sets, the cast may be polished with wet hands to ensure a smooth finish.

Finally, all excess plaster should be removed and the surrounding skin dried before the patient is allowed to leave.

Preparing Slabs

Slabs are used for strengthening areas of potential weakness and for reducing the weight of large casts. They may be prepared either by unrolling a Gypsona bandage to the required length and folding it into 5 or 6 layers, or by withdrawing the required length of 5-ply bandages from a Gypsona plaster slab dispenser. When the required length (plus 10 % to allow for shrinkage) and width have been decided, the slab is lightly folded from each end to the centre. After immersion in a bucket of cool water (25-85°C) the slab is immediately removed and carefully and quickly smoothed out on a flat surface, or held in one hand

and the fingers of the other hand drawn down the slab. The use of cooler water lengthens the setting time. To ensure that this results in a strong homogeneous cast, the layers must be compressed together and the bubbles excluded. For convenience of handling and application, the smoothed slab should then be lightly folded again.

Care of the Wet Cast

Until a cast is fully dry, it is liable to be damaged by pressure.

The completed wet cast should be handled with care and correctly supported to protect it from damage. A plaster cast takes 3 to 5 minutes to set, depending on its thickness and the temperature of the water used for soaking the bandage. However, the time required for a cast to dry **varies** according to its type and position. For example, a forearm plaster will dry in 36 hours, a leg plaster in 48 hours and trunk plasters or plaster beds may not be wholly dry for 72 hours, depending on the atmospheric conditions. When tapped gently with the knuckles, a wet cast will emit a dull sound, whereas the sound from a dry cast will be crisp and clear.

While drying is in progress concave parts of the cast should be supported to prevent pressure on convex parts. This rule applies regardless of the type of plaster or the posture of the patient. Ambulant patients with upper limb casts should wear a sling until the plaster is dry. If a lower limb cast has been applied, the patient should remain immobile or be supplied with crutches, otherwise unavoidable pressure will be put on the wet cast, causing softening of the sole.

Instructions for the Patient

A patient who is sent home wearing a plaster cast should receive both verbal and written instructions on the care of the cast. The latter should be on a printed card. It is imperative that the patient fully understands these instructions; it is not sufficient merely to hand over an instruction card and rapidly read it to the patient who, because of his or her condition or the effect of the hospital surroundings, may be somewhat confused. The only way to ensure that the patient fully understands the instructions and will co-operate is to go over the points one by one, explaining their importance. Instructions for a child in a cast would be given to the parent or guardian. With older children, it is useful to explain the instructions to them as well to assist the parents in gaining their full co-operation. For elderly patients and for patients who are confined to bed at home, the nurse would advise those caring for them or would organize professional assistance.

The patient should be instructed on how to maintain muscle tone and keep swelling to a minimum by exercising the extremities of the damaged limb. Any written instructions on these exercises should be augmented by demonstrations from the nurse. The patient should then be asked to perform the exercises, to make sure that the instructions are fully understood. This will also establish whether the cast restricts movement in any way. See pp. 248-9, 254-5 and 259.

Complications

Swelling

Some swelling accompanies every fracture; it is likely to be substantially more severe whenever reduction is performed. It is vital, therefore, that the nurse should anticipate any such swelling by applying a suitably padded cast. It is essential that the damaged limb should be kept elevated and that the extremities are exercised during the 24 hours subsequent to the cast being applied.

As the swelling subsides during the first 2 days, a cast can become loose. For this reason, initial immobilization with a plaster slab may be preferable to a full cast which can be applied later, e.g., with a Colles's fracture (see later section).

Plaster Sores

Plaster sores may develop for a number of reasons. They may result from poor technique, inadequate instructions to the patient, lack of postcasting supervision or foreign bodies.

Poor Technique. Poor technique could involve:
    Lumpiness in the completed cast.
    Inadequate skeletal protection by padding.
    Failure to trim the extremities of the cast.
    A cast that fits poorly around bony prominences.

Inadequate Instructions for the Patient. As a result of inadequate instructions to the patient from the nurse, a patient may fail to understand how to care for the cast properly. This can lead to the development of uneven pressure, friction, wetting and cracking of the cast, with inevitable skin damage.

Lack of Postcasting Supervision. As a part of postcasting supervision, it is imperative for the nurse to take note of patient's who complain of pain under their casts, particularly when the pain does not emanate from the site of injury. Ischaemic skin or severe pain in the limb is most commonly caused by points of excessive tightness or looseness in a cast. Pain can result either directly from local pressure or indirectly from arterial occlusion which in itself could be caused by a poorly fitting cast. Regardless of the cause, investigation should be immediate and appropriate corrective measures should be taken without delay.

Foreign Bodies. A serious complication can occur when a foreign body is introduced either intentionally or accidentally between the plaster cast and the skin.

1 Young children wearing plaster casts should be strictly supervised to prevent them hiding small toys, coins or sweets inside the cast. Should such items come to rest in a closely fitting section of the cast, they may cause the development of severe sores.

2 All patients should be advised not to scratch the skin beneath the cast, particularly with metal implements, e.g., knitting needles, back scratchers. Apart from disturbing the padding, scratching can damage the skin, resulting in the development of infected sores. If these are suspected then an inspection window should be cut in the cast. After inspection, the window should be replaced and bandaged in position. If this is not done oedema will develop within the windowed area, leading to soreness of the skin at the margins of the cut square.

3 Special consideration should always be given to the patient who has a lower limb plaster in which a window has been cut since the weight-bearing ability of the cast is significantly reduced. The alternative to cutting a window is to bivalve the cast which enables a more extensive inspection to be carried out, but once the situation has been ascertained, a replacement cast will be necessary.

Loss of Power

Apart from nerve damage caused at the time of injury, loss of power, such as the inability to extend the fingers or toes, can result from:
- Pressure of the plaster on a superficial nerve — the padding of vulnerable points can reduce the danger of nerve damage.
- Prolonged tourniquet pressure postoperatively.
- Impaired arterial flow — may be a complication of the injury or subsequent swelling.

Sensation and the power of the extremities should be checked frequently after the application of a cast and any impairment or loss in power should be investigated immediately. If either of the first 2 points listed above are believed to be the cause, then the tension may be relieved by splitting the cast. To prevent overstretching of weak muscles, the fingers and toes may be supported by adding on a plaster platform. In all cases, the action taken will depend on the situation, but gentle, active exercises should be undertaken to assist circulation and strengthen muscles; if active movement is not possible, then passive exercise should be encouraged.

Impaired Circulation

Impaired Venous Return

Blueness and swelling of the extremeties of the damaged limb suggest that the venous return is impaired because of the tightness of the plaster. The blueness of venous congestion must be differentiated from bruising. For example, extensive bruising of the digits is a feature of a Colles' fracture that has been reduced manually. Normal circulation in the damaged limb is checked by pinching a toe or finger nail which should immediately flush pink when the pressure is relieved. If venous return is sluggish, the limb should be elevated and digital exercises should be performed as vigorously as possible. This action is usually all that is required. If the situation persists, however, and the patient is experiencing discomfort the cast should be split, eased, and then held firmly in place with a cotton bandage. Splitting may be carried out by using an electric cutter, the combination of a small plaster handsaw and a plaster knife, or plaster shears. The cut should be made on the lateral aspect of the cast, following a line marked down its length. Splitting may be done as a routine postoperative procedure or in the event of unrelieved circulatory impairment.

Impaired Arterial Flow

Impaired arterial flow is usually associated with the injury that has necessitated immobilization. Because it demands urgent medical attention, it is imperative that it be recognized early in the course of treatment.

Signs and Symptoms. The signs and symptoms of impaired arterial flow include:
    Pallor of affected area of skin
    Increasing pain
    Lack of pulse distal to the injury
    Loss of power
When the radial pulse is covered by a plaster cast, normal arterial flow in the damaged limb may be demonstrated by pinching the finger nail which should immediately flush pink.

The temperature of the digits should also be noted, since cold digits indicate an impaired arterial flow.

Action. Medical advice should be obtained immediately. Splitting the cast may relieve the pressure of an arterial haematoma but if the artery has gone into spasm, surgical intervention may be required.

Instructions for the Patient

To maintain general fitness during the period of immobilization, patients should be instructed to exercise those parts of the body not encased in plaster.
The main benefits from this are:
    Joints are kept mobile — stiffness related to inactivity is prevented.
    Musculature is kept in good tone — rehabilitation is greatly assisted by muscle control.
    Complications of deep venous thrombosis, coronary or pulmonary infarction will be reduced — if the general circulation is maintained through an exercise programme which should include deep-breathing exercises.

Slab for a New Colles's Fracture

To apply a slab for a new Colles's fracture the arm is positioned as in Figure 65a. Remove all rings from the patient's fingers. The plaster will extend from the metacarpal heads to just below the elbow crease. Ensure that there is no restriction to flexion of the finger or elbow joints.

Application

To apply a slab for a Colles's fracture:
1 Apply stockinette and allow for a 3 cm turnover at each end of the cast. Make a hole for the thumb (Figure 65b).
2 Apply padding around the wrist and upper forearm (Figure 65c). Padding may be applied in the form of Orthoban covering the stockinette.

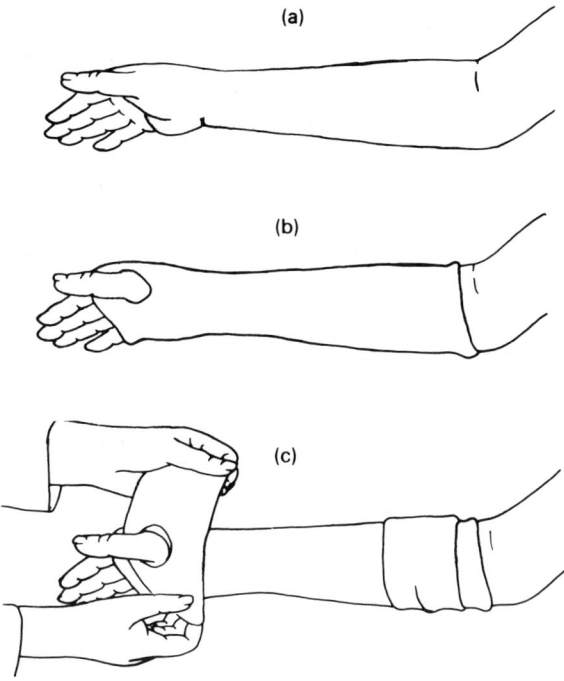

Figure 65 Application of a slab for a new Colles's fracture: place the arm in the correct position (a); apply stockinette making a hole for the thumb (b); apply padding around the wrist and upper forearm (c).

3 Measure the length of slab required (Figure 65d) and check the circumference of the arm. The slab should encompass two thirds of the circumference of the forearm.

4 Cut the length of the slab required either from a slab dispenser or make up from 5 layers of Gypsona bandage and shape as necessary (Figure 65e).

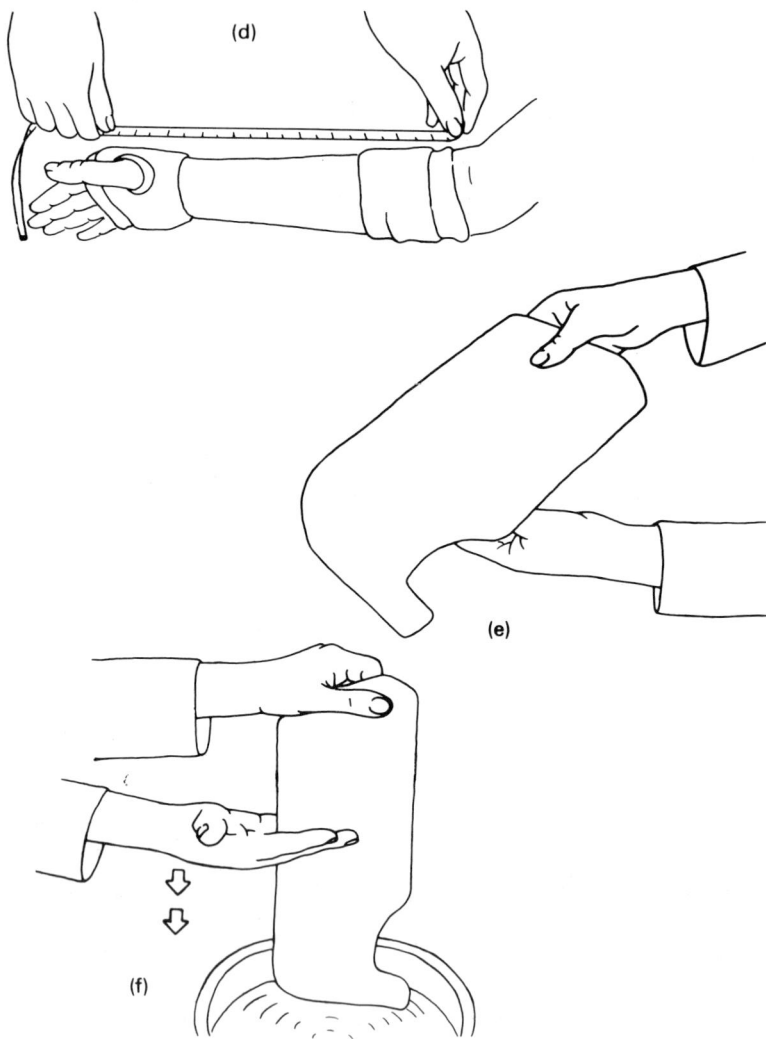

Figure 65 (cont.) Measure the length of the slab required (d); prepare the slab (e); emerse slab in water and then expel surplus water (f).

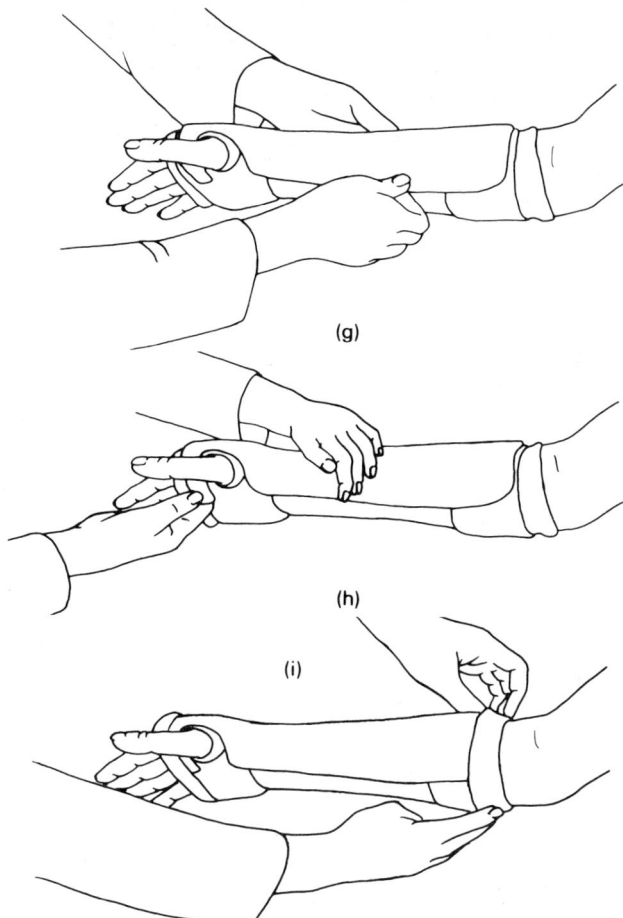

Figure 65 (cont.) Position the slab on the arm (g); mould the slab to the shape of the arm (h); trim edge and turn stockinette or padding over the ends of the slab (i).

5 Hold the slab by the ends and immerse in water. Draw fingers down the slab to expel surplus water (Figure 65f).

6 Position the slab on the arm around the ventral surface of the radius and base of the first metacarpal (Figure 65g). Ensure that the limb is in the correct position to maintain alignment of the fractured bone.

7 Mould the slab with the flat side of your hands (Figure 65h).

8 Trim back if there is any restriction to flexion of the joints. Turn back the stockinette or padding over the ends of the slab (Figure 65i).

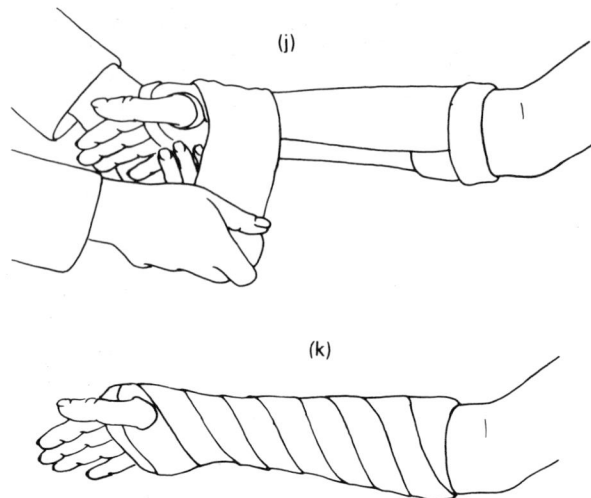

Figure 65 (cont.) Apply a wet Crinx or gauze bandage (j); complete the application of the bandage (k).

9 Apply a wet Crinx or gauze bandage to hold the slab in position against the hand and forearm (Figure 65j). Retain the end of the bandage with a soaked piece of waste slab material. Alternatively a crepe bandage may be used to hold the slab in position.
10 Finish off the cast as shown in Figure 65k and clean off splashes of plaster from the patient's skin with a damp cloth.
11 Support the arm in a sling. The splint will be converted into a complete cast in 24 hours or as soon as the swelling has subsided. Instruct the patient regarding exercises for the fingers, elbow and shoulder joints, and give advice regarding care of the plaster and when to return to the clinic.

Completing the Colles's Plaster

To complete the Colles's plaster:
1 Cut through the Crinx or gauze bandage (Figure 66a) or remove crepe bandage; check if the plaster slab is fitting correctly. If it is not fitted, remove carefully and make another one.
2 Soak and apply a 7.5 cm wide Gypsona bandage around the

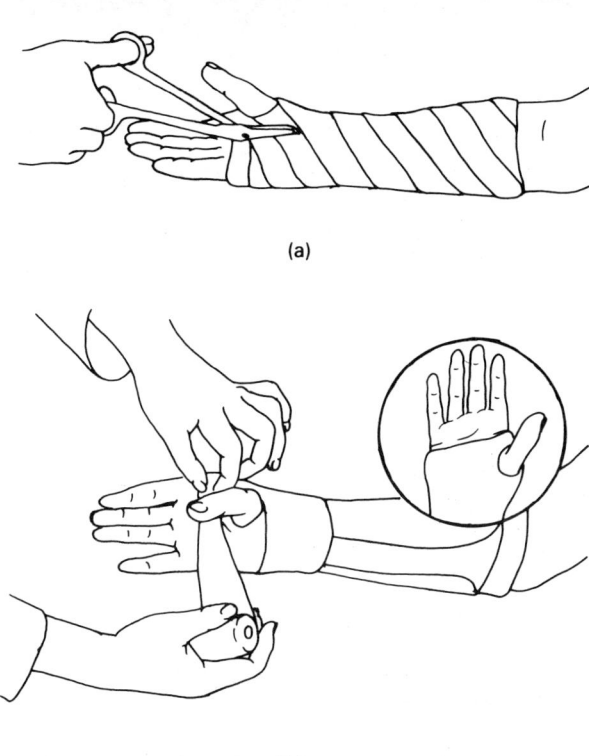

Figure 66 Completing the Colles's plaster: cut through the Crinx or gauze bandage to check if the plaster is fitting correctly (a); apply a Gypsona bandage around the wrist and hand making sure the band of plaster over the web of the thumb is as narrow as possible (b, and insert).

wrist and hand (Figure 66b), making sure that the band of plaster over the web of the thumb is as narrow as possible (Figure 66b, insert). If the stockinette has been applied, turn over the edge on the first turn of the plaster and secure by the second turn leaving a soft edge. The edge of the plaster must not extend beyond the horizontal crease of the palm otherwise the metacarpophalangeal joints will be restricted.

3 Continue along the arm (Figure 66c), overlapping turns by half the width of the bandage.

4 Soak a 10 cm wide Gypsona bandage and apply from the top of the plaster (Figure 66d) folding over and securing the stockinette as previously described.

5 Mould around the limb in a circular motion using the flats of your hands (Figure 66e).

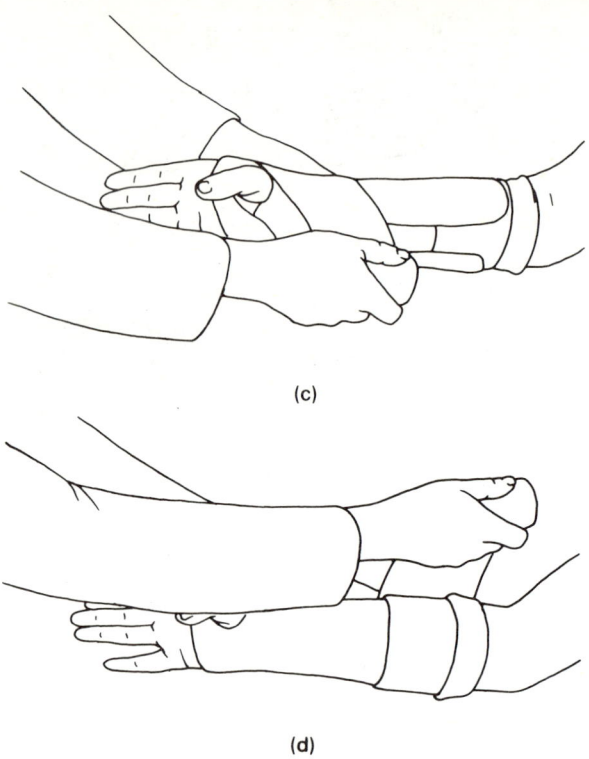

Figure 66 (cont.) Continue applying the bandage along the arm (c); apply another Gypsona bandage from the top of the plaster (d).

6 Ensure the patient is able to flex the finger (Figure 66f) and elbow joints. Clean off splashes of plaster from the patient's skin with a damp cloth. Apply a sling for the first 24 hours or until the plaster has set.

Instructions for the Patient

1 While your cast is still wet (depending on the material used this may be up to 36 hours), it is especially important not to knock, dent or further wet your plaster. Do not rest your arm on any hard object as this may dent the plaster.
2 Keep the injured arm elevated in a sling. When sitting or in bed keep the arm elevated on a pillow with the hand above the level of the heart.
3 Gently exercise the finger joints and also the elbow and shoulder joints of the injured arm.

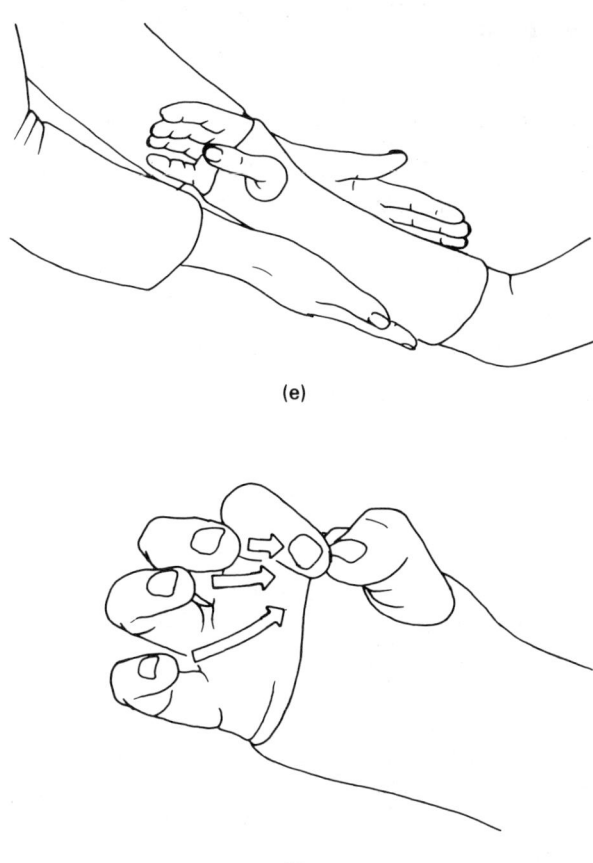

(e)

(f)

Figure 66 (cont.) Mould the bandage to the shape of the limb (e); ensure that there is no restriction to flexion of the fingers (f). The finger movement shown (f) is also an exercise.

4   Ensure that there is a suitable analgesic available. Aspirin or paracetamol are usually effective. There will be some pain but it should subside. If the pain becomes more severe, if there is a change in skin colour of the fingers to white or blue, or if there is alteration of sensation in the fingers, e.g., 'pins and needles' or numbness, then return immediately to the department or to the local doctor.
5   Do not put any objects under your plaster, e.g., paper, coins.
6   If the plaster becomes loose or cracked report to the hospital as soon as possible.

Below-knee Plaster

Before applying a below-the-knee plaster, the patient's foot is positioned at a 90° angle to the leg and neutral to inversion and eversion. The affected leg is placed over a knee rest with the toes in line with the knee (Figure 67a). The plaster will extend from the metatarsophalangeal joints to a point just below the head of the fibula.

Application

To apply a below-the-knee plaster:
1 Apply a stockinette, allowing for a turn at each end of the cast (Figure 67b).
2 Apply padding, e.g., Orthoban, as required but particularly around the malleoli and the upper part of the leg and over the shin (Figure 67c) or continuously from the metatarsophalangeal joint to below the head of the fibula.
3 Measure the length of the back slab from the base of the toes, under the foot, around the heel and up the leg level with a point just below the head of the fibula and add 7.5 – 10 cm. The back slab should extend under the foot to the metatarsal heads and the end turned back to give double strength for the foot. Lateral cuts should be made in the slab of the heel to allow for a smooth fitting at the corner. Measure a slab from just below the head of the fibula on the anterior aspect of the leg to the base of the toes allowing 5 cm extra for shrinkage. Cut a 15 cm slab for the first mentioned and a 10 cm wide slab for the second (Figure 67d). These may be either cut from a slab dispenser or made up from Gypsona bandages 5 layers thick.
4 Commence construction of the cast by soaking and applying the 15 cm slab posteriorly and the 10 cm slab anteriorly to the leg (Figure 67e).
5 Continue construction of the cast by soaking and applying a 15 cm Gypsona bandage from below the fibula head to the ankle (Figure 67f).
6 Complete construction of the cast by applying another 15 cm bandage from the ankle to the metatarsal heads (Figure 67g).
7 Mould and smooth to the contours of the limb with the flats of your hands (Figure 67h), particularly around the malleoli. Find the roots of the toes and mould plaster to reform the transverse arch. Ensure that the position of the limb has been maintained.

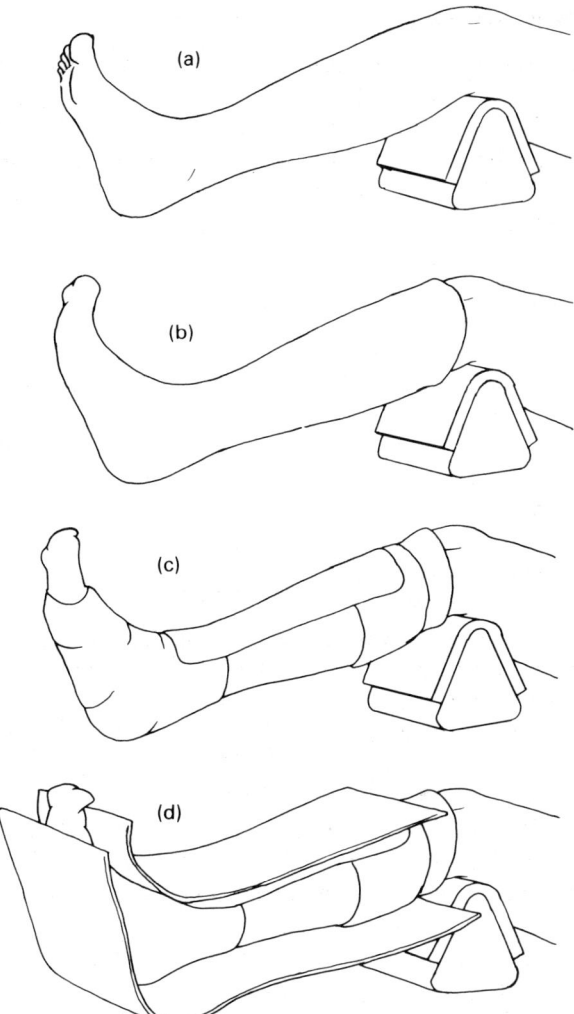

Figure 67 Application of a below-knee plaster: place the leg in the correct position (a); apply stockinette (b); apply padding as required, particularly around the malleoli and upper part of the leg (c); measure two slabs for above and below the leg (d).

8 Trim where necessary, ensuring that the little toe can be seen and that there is freedom of movement for the toes and full knee flexion without restriction. Fold back the stockinette at both ends (Figure 67i).

9 Apply two 15 cm Gypsona bandages to secure the slabs and

to finish off the cast (Figure 67j). Smooth the cast with the flats of your hands. Clean off splashes of plaster from the patient's skin. If a walking plaster is required, the sole will be protected by a fitting of a Böhler iron, a wooden or rubber walking appliance, or a canvas boot.

10 Issue crutches with instructions if required (see Chapter 4).

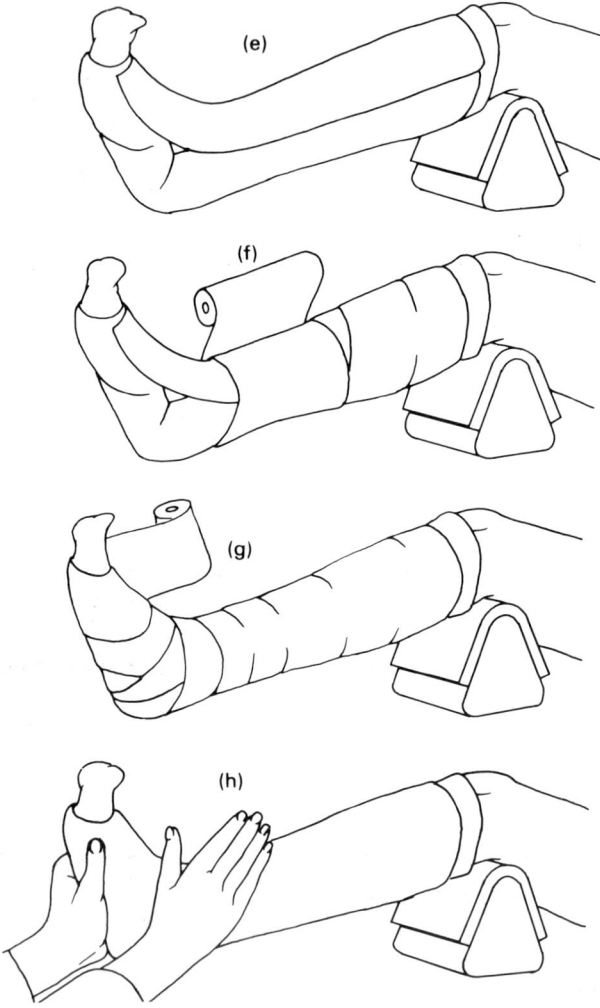

Figure 67 (cont.) Soak and apply the slabs (e); soak and apply another Gypsona bandage from below the fibula head to the ankle (f); apply the final Gypsona bandage from the ankle to the metatarsal head (g); mould and smooth to the contours of the limb (h).

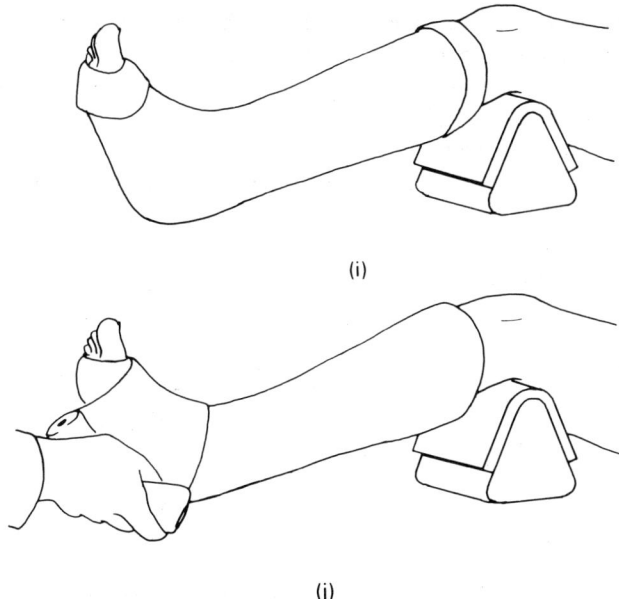

Figure 67 (cont.) Trim where necessary and fold back stockinette at both ends (i); apply two bandages to secure slabs and to finish off the cast (j).

Instructions for the Patient

1 While your cast is still wet and this may be up to 48 hours depending on the material used, it is essential that you do not knock, dent or further wet your plaster.
2 Do not bear weight on your leg until the plaster is dry. You may be issued with crutches.
3 Do not rest your leg on any hard objects as this will dent your plaster.
4 Do not put any objects between your skin and the plaster, e.g., paper, coins.
5 Keep your leg elevated on a stool with a pillow keeping the foot above knee level while sitting.
6 Exercise all joints not included in the plaster especially:
   Toes movements
   Extension and flexion of the knee joint
   Circular movement of the hip joint
7 If the plaster becomes loose or cracked report to the hospital as soon as possible.
8 If your toes become swollen, more painful, change in colour

from pint to white, mottled or blue, or feel like 'pins and needles', return to the doctor or hospital immediately.

REVISION OBJECTIVES

1 Identify the problems related to head and face injuries and comment upon the psychological and physical care.
2 State the cause and effect of injuries to the chest.
3 Describe the treatment of injuries to the lungs and patient care during the insertion of a chest drain.
4 List the cause of abdominal injuries and the organs or structures that may be affected describing the signs, symptoms, patient care and treatment.
5 List the structures that may be damaged with pelvic injuries and describe the patient care with special reference to the moving of the patient and observations of urinary output.
6 ·Identify and describe the types of fracture.
7 Detail the signs and symptoms of a suspected fracture and elaborate upon immediate patient care.
8 Describe the treatment of common fractures.
9 List the methods of sedation and appropriate patient care involved in the reduction of a fracture.
10 Explain the effects of spinal, pelvic and limb injuries.
11 Illustrate the application of skin traction and a Thomas' splint.
12 List the complications of a fracture.
13 Apply a plaster of Paris and advise a patient regarding care on discharge.

10
Surgical and Gynaecological Emergencies

Many patients are referred to the accident and emergency department for further investigation when there is the possibility of surgery being required to alleviate the problem. These patients may present with an acute condition, which is abdominal or gynaecological in nature.

ACUTE ABDOMINAL CONDITIONS

An acute abdominal condition can arise from a variety of causes but may present with similar characteristics.

Signs and Symptoms

Characteristic signs of an acute abdominal condition:
- Sudden onset
- Pain — The pain may be continuous or spasmodic, diffuse or specific.
- Progress — swift deterioration.

Other signs and symptoms which may accompany an acute abdominal condition:
- Nausea
- Vomiting
- Constipation
- Diarrhoea
- Abdominal distension
- Rigid, flat abdominal wall
- Anxiety
- Shock

Causes

The cause of the acute abdominal condition is varied and the effect depends on the organ or structure involved. It can be caused by foreign material, inflammation, obstruction or haemorrhage.

Irritant foreign material within the peritoneal cavity will result from a perforation or rupture of any structure causing leakage of contents into the cavity.

Inflammatory causes are due usually to chemical or bacterial action.

Obstruction of any tract within the abdomen. This will include renal, biliary or alimentary tract obstructions and vascular obstructions such as strangulations. It can be due to neurogenic failure and part of the bowel may have stopped functioning, e.g., after traumatic injury caused by severe crushing.

Haemorrhage due to damage to the blood vessels from disease or trauma or by a disorder of the blood vessels, e.g., abdominal aortic aneurysm.

Patient Care

For care of the patient, it is necessary to support the patient on a trolley in a position of comfort taking consideration of the patient's general needs to prevent further complications.

To obtain **comfort** the patient may ease the pain by curling up on one side or lying on his or her back with knees bent. However some patients may find difficulty in obtaining relief of pain in any position. If the patient is restless make sure that the sides of the trolley are fastened up securely to prevent the patient falling out.

According to the **general condition** of the patient, a loss of fluid from the circulatory system, as a result of either vomiting or haemorrhage, will leave the patient in a condition of hypovolaemia. Keep the patient in a recumbent position to ensure that the blood is circulating to the vital organs.

To prevent **further complications,** if the blood pressure is not decreased, the patient may be nursed in semirecumbent position to relieve any respiratory difficulty.

Nausea and vomiting often accompany acute abdominal conditions so make sure that the patient has a vomit bowl and tissues.

Ensure that the patient's airway is not obstructed and that if there is vomiting, the vomitus is not inhaled. Position the patient upright or on one side to prevent this happening.

Use suction apparatus if necessary to remove vomitus from the patient's airway.
If the patient vomits observe, report and record the results.
Allow the patient a mouthwash to clean the mouth.
Do **not** give the patient anything by mouth and make sure that the patient and the relatives or friends understand this. A nasogastric tube may be passed to remove gastric contents and to allow the gastrointestinal tract to rest.
The patient with an acute abdomen will require an intravenous infusion. This will replace:
  Blood loss from haemorrhage.
  Fluid loss from vomiting. The patient who has vomited will also require the addition of electrolytes to maintain the balance of electrolytes within the body. Normal range for sodium 135–145 mmol litre^{-1} and for potassium 3.5–5.0 mmol litre^{-1}.

Assessment

The following observations should be recorded every 15 minutes for an assessment of the patient's condition:
1 Blood pressure and pulse to observe for the condition of shock. The pulse may be elevated if the patient has pyrexia.
2 Respirations.
3 Temperature — this may be elevated in conditions of inflammation or infection.
4 Any vomitus or diarrhoea must be observed for:
  Colour — haematemesis, melaena.
  Consistency —
    Vomitus — watery or like coffee grounds.
    Diarrhoea — sticky or tarry.
  Amount — this must be recorded.
5 Urine must be tested. Urine should also be saved to be sieved to observe for renal calculi if the doctor suspects renal colic as a possible diagnosis of the patient's condition.

Pain

The patient's history is essential for the doctor to have in order to make a diagnosis. The intensity and location of pain provide an excellent indication of the cause and seriousness of the condition. Observe and listen carefully to the patient as the pain is described.

The patient may point to the site of the pain or place a hand over the abdomen which could indicate diffuse (generalized) pain. The patient may describe the pain as continuous, intermittent, sharp, dull, or burning. In some cases the patient may have complained of pain and then the pain is suddenly relieved.

Observe the abdomen of the patient. The abdomen may be rigid and flat, looking and feeling as hard as a board and, whilst the patient is not feeling any pain, the abdominal muscles may be reacting to an acute situation within the abdomen. This is often the case in peritonitis due to a perforation.

Observe the patient for other signs and symptoms, expecially shock and pyrexia.

The patient will not receive analgesia until the pain has been assessed by the doctor. Analgesia will reduce the patient's awareness of pain and in some conditions, especially a suspected condition, the doctor will rely on continuous accurate reports of pain. Increasing pain usually indicates the need for surgery. The analgesia which is usually given is a controlled drug, e.g., papaveretum. Remember analgesia will have the effect of depressing the central nervous system causing drowsiness and may decrease the respiratory rate.

Types of Pain. The pain may be generalized, spasmodic or continuous.

Generalized burning in inflammatory conditions may localize later to an actual area, e.g., right iliac fossa — appendicitis.

Spasmodic pain (colic) — The pain of increased peristaltic action generally due to an obstruction.

Continuous severe pain due to *ischaemia*, loss of blood supply to part of the abdominal contents, e.g., strangulated hernia.

Diagnostic Tests

X-ray

Abdominal X-rays (erect and supine) are taken to observe for gas and fluid levels in the abdomen. A routine chest X-ray is also taken.

The taking of X-rays can often involve long waits for the patient and can be an uncomfortable procedure as the patient is required to move into various positions. Some accident and emergency departments are fortunate enough to have their own or very closely attached X-ray departments while other hospitals necessitate the patient being taken to the X-ray department, usually along a draughty corridor.

When a patient in an acute situation requires an X-ray:

1 Always ensure that a qualified nurse accompanies the patient. Nurse learners in an accident and emergency department will be unused to dealing with an acutely ill patient and may become anxious when expected to attend to one. It is important for nurse learners to be assisted during their short stay in the department, as they are there to learn, so they should be able to say when they are not happy about accompanying a patient. There are situations which worry everyone, including trained staff, but an apprehensive nurse is not able to meet fully the psychological and physical needs of the patient. This is why careful decisions are made in the allocation of jobs when it is at all possible.

2 Ensure that the X-ray department is expecting and is ready to take the patient immediately.

3 Ensure that the patient is warm enough. Take an extra blanket if necessary.

4 If the patient requires any treatment make sure either that this is given before the patient goes to the X-ray department or that the accompanying nurse takes the appropriate equipment, e.g., intravenous fluid if the intravenous infusion will require changing while the patient is in X-ray.

5 Assist the patient to move to the correct position for the X-ray with the help of the radiographer.

6 The nurse must know the location of the emergency equipment within the X-ray department.

7 If the patient is not acutely ill and a nurse is not needed to be in attendance then inform the waiting relative or friend to accompany and stay with the patient.

Blood Tests

All blood samples will be taken before intravenous fluids are administered. Above normal levels of leucocytes (normal 4 – 11 $\times\ 10^9$ litre $^{-1}$) will indicate inflammation. Above normal levels of serum amylase will indicate disease of the pancreas. The patient who has a haemorrhage will have decreased haemoglobin and may require blood transfusion.

Electrocardiogram

An electrocardiogram will be taken to assess the heart's function especially in those patients preparing for theatre.

Urine Tests

A mid-stream urine specimen may be sent to confirm a urinary tract infection or bleeding.

Rectal Examination

Gynaecological History and Examination

Gynaecological conditions in women of child-bearing age can present as an acute abdomen. The pain a woman can complain of at the time of ovulation in the menstrual cycle may mimic the pain of an inflammatory condition. Inflammation of the uterine tubes (salpingitis) may also present as an acute abdomen. A gynaecological condition which produces an acute abdominal emergency is an ectopic pregnancy (see p. 268).

Inflammation

Inflammatory conditions may affect several parts of the lower abdomen, e.g., cholecystitis, pancreatitis, diverticulitis.

Treatment

Treatment is usually conservative allowing rest until the inflammation has subsided. Treatment involves:
1. Nil by mouth
2. Nasogastric tube with aspiration
3. Intravenous therapy
4. Bed rest
5. Frequent observation or assessment of:
   Temperature
   Pulse
   Blood pressure
   Respirations
   Pain
6. Antibiotic therapy if indicated
7. Antiemetic and analgesic drugs if ordered.

Haemorrhage

An *aneurysm*, a dilatation of an artery, due to weakness of the arterial wall may lead to the rupture of the artery and haemorrhage.

Treatment

Treatment will involve surgery to repair the artery.

Obstruction

Obstructions of the bowel can be divided into 2 groups which both present with their similar signs and symptoms but there are important differences in their treatment.
    Subacute — incomplete obstruction
    Acute — complete obstruction

Causes

The causes of subacute and acute obstructions are similar:

Growths can occur either within the bowel or cause pressure from without. A cause of blockage within the bowel is hard impacted faeces. A cause of blockage from outside the bowel may be adhesions. This is when fibrous bands form in some cases after abdominal surgery.

Inflammatory conditions include diverticulitis which is an inflammation of a diverticulum, a small pouch formed by the mucosal lining of the bowel pushing through the muscle layer to form a sac outside the bowel. This condition usually affects the descending colon. Stagnation of bowel contents within the diverticulum lead to an inflammatory reaction causing local swelling and may cause obstruction of the bowel.

Abnormal positions of the bowel can lead to:
    Hernia — the protrusion of the bowel through the peritoneal lining.
    Volvulus — twisting of part of the intestines.
    Intussusception — part of the intestines pushes into the part next to it; this usually occurs in children.

Damage to the nerve supply to the bowel may lead to non-functioning of the bowel producing a *paralytic ileus*. The obstruction occurs here because the peristalic action is no longer present and so the contents cannot be moved through this section.

Treatment

Subacute Conditions. A subacute condition may be treated conservatively, as in inflammatory conditions. A patient with a subacute obstruction may be given an enema in an attempt to remove the obstruction, e.g., impacted faeces.

Acute Conditions. With an acute condition, the patient is taken for surgery to relieve the obstruction. If the obstruction is to the arterial supply, as in a strangulated hernia, when an organ has pushed through the muscle wall of its lining and due to the muscle constriction has lost its blood supply, then immediate surgery is required to relieve the obstruction and to prevent gangrene of the affected area.

GYNAECOLOGICAL CONDITIONS

Gynaecological conditions are quite frequently seen in the accident and emergency department. Abdominal pain in women between the ages of fourteen and sixty are frequently due to gynaecological problems. One of the most serious acute conditions is the ectopic pregnancy. Other problems include pain, infection and haemorrhage.

Unfortunately, the cause of many women attending an accident and emergency department is due to a complication of pregnancy. This may mean that the woman has a physical condition that must be given psychological consideration because of the circumstances that have brought her to the department.

Ectopic Pregnancy

The word ectopic is Greek and means 'out of place' so an *ectopic* pregnancy is a pregnancy which is not within the uterus.

The ovum leaves the ovary, passes through the small section of the pelvic cavity to enter the uterine, or fallopian, tube. Once within the uterine tube the ovum is moved towards the uterus. During the movement along the uterine tube the ovum, for pregnancy to occur, must be fertilized by a sperm. This becomes the zygote and normally embeds itself in the wall of the uterus. In the case of an ectopic pregnancy the zygote embeds itself in the uterine tube or the pelvic cavity. The zygote may be unable to obtain sufficient nourishment and therefore dies. This may present a nagging pain for which the patient may not require any hospital treatment as the zygote is gradually absorbed.

The serious problem with th ectopic pregnancy is when the zygote embeds itself within the uterine tube and its growth eventually perforates the tube. The contents are then dispersed into the peritoneal cavity causing peritonitis.

The patient may come to the accident and emergency department with a lower abdominal pain, before the time of the perforation. A diagnosis of this condition and the removal of the zygote from the uterine tube by surgery can prevent the problems of a ruptured ectopic pregnancy. The problems being haemorrhage and peritonitis. The rupture of the uterine tube involves tearing the blood vessels to which the zygote is attached. The patient will be in a condition of shock and will require immediate treatment.

Psychological Effect

Another important consideration is the psychological effect upon the patient. The patient is generally only 3 - 6 weeks pregnant when the ectopic pregnancy ruptures and may not even have been aware of the pregnancy if there was no change in the menstrual cycle. However, the suddenness of onset, the pain and the thought that she could have been pregnant can be very upsetting to the patient. Allow the patient to talk about it if she wishes and contact and allow her partner to visit if possible in the short time that will be available before surgery.

Treatment

The surgery will involve a salpingectomy, the removal of the affected uterine tube and drainage of foreign material from the abdomen.

Apart from the treatment for shock and preparation for theatre while in the accident and emergency department, the patient may be given antibiotic therapy before surgery to prevent the complication of peritonitis.

Inflammation

Salpingitis is an inflammatory condition of the uterine tubes. This condition has been mentioned in the section on the acute abdomen (see p. 266) as the signs and symptoms are very similar. Treatment is conservative once other conditions such as an ectopic pregnancy have been ruled out.

Pregnancy Irregularities

With irregularities in a normal pregnancy the general practitioner is usually contacted first. These irregularities may be bleeding or pain.

Care and treatment is aimed at preventing the loss of the pregnancy. *Abortion* is the loss of the fetus before the twentieth week of gestation. After the twentieth week until the expected delivery date the fetus will be considered as *premature*. Both abortion and premature delivery bring patients into the accident and emergency department.

Classification of Abortion

Abortion can be classified as:
    Complete — when all the contents are discharged.
    Incomplete — when some of the contents remain.
    Missed — when all previous signs of pregnancy disappear and the uterus eventually discharges a blood clot with the remains of the fetus (*carneous mole*).
    Inevitable — there may be severe vaginal bleeding. The uterus contracts, resulting in abdominal pain and the cervix

Presenting Situation

The presenting situation for abortion is:
    Threatened — This is characterized by bleeding during pregnancy and abdominal pain. The cervix **may be** dilated.
    Inevitable — there may be severe vaginal bleeding. The uterus contracts, resulting in abdominal pain and the cervix **is** dilated. The fetus is expelled.
    Spontaneous — The uterine contents are expelled completely and normally, before the twentieth week.

Induced Abortion

Abortions can be induced and are classified as therapeutic or criminal. For a **therapeutic** abortion, the patient will not come to the accident and emergency department, as the abortion is arranged and conducted in hospital by the doctor due to the mother's health status.

A **criminal** abortion is an attempt to remove the fetus by an unqualified person or persons. Since the abortion act (1967) in the United Kingdom the number of criminal abortions has decreased.

Complications of a criminal abortion can be:
 Incomplete evacuation
 Perforation of the uterus
 Severe haemorrhage
 Generalized infection — septicaemia, due to insterile technique.

The signs and symptoms for a criminal abortion may include abdominal pain and blood loss or foul-smelling blood-stained discharge per vagina.

Assessment

The immediate condition must be assessed and treated:
1 Observation of blood pressure and pulse will indicate whether the patient is in a condition of shock. If so the patient must be treated appropriately (see Chapter 3).
2 Observations of vaginal blood loss must be maintained. The patient's sanitary pads must be observed and changed regularly noting blood loss.
3 Observations of temperature must be maintained, reported and recorded.
4 Observations of pain, noting its severity and frequency, will denote the uterine contractions. Administration of analgesia when ordered by the doctor.

Doctor's Examination. Most departments now have a gynaecologist on call to examine and treat patients with gynaecological conditions. This prevents the patient being subjected to unnecessary examination. The examination includes:
1 An accurate obstetric history.

2   A vaginal examination. A dilated cervix will conclude that the abortion is inevitable.

Patient Care

Remember the psychological care of the patient. The nurse must prepare and remain with the patient during the doctor's examination. Provide explanations and reassurance as this will aid in calming the patient. Also ensure that the patient has privacy.

Treatment

The aim of treatment is to preserve the pregnancy if at all possible so the patient must be placed on a trolley to rest.

Threatened. Treatment of a patient with a threatened abortion:
1   Rest — the patient is often admitted to hospital.
2   Observations of pain and vaginal loss.

Spontaneous, Inevitable and Incomplete. Treatment for a spontaneous, inevitable or incomplete abortion:
1   Hospital admission.
2   Ergometrine maleate may be given to control the bleeding following abortion.
   Oxytocin (Syntometrine) may be given to induce labour and therefore aid evacuation of the uterus. This must be given by slow intravenous infusion.
3   Operation of dilatation and curettage to remove any possible remains with the uterus.
Remember:
   The patient may have suffered a severe haemorrhage.
   The patient may be in need of psychological care.

Criminal or Septic. Treatment for a criminal or septic abortion involves hospital admission.
Treatment involves:
1   Intravenous infusion — to aid in correction of shock
2   Antibiotics — to prevent or treat infection
3   Regular observations of blood pressure, pulse, respirations, temperature and vaginal loss.
4   Analgesia for pain.

5 A dilatation and curettage when the patient's condition has improved.

Eclampsia

Eclampsia is a condition which occurs in pregnancy after the twenty-eighth week. It is due to poisoning of the blood by the absorption of toxins and occurs in 2 stages:
   Pre-eclampsia — a percursor of eclampsia
   Eclampsia
Both conditions require hospital treatment.

Signs and Symptoms

Signs and symptoms of eclampsia include:
   Hypertension
   Oedemia
   Proteinuria
   Headaches
   Vomiting and abdominal pain
   Oliguria
A complication of this condition may result in a fit and this may be the reason why the patient has come to the accident and emergency department (see Chapter 8). Important considerations:
1 Maintain airway
2 Summon obstetric personnel
   Once the patient's fit has been controlled she will be admitted for further treatment to the obstetric department.

Obstetric Emergencies

Obstetric emergencies may occur before the thirty-sixth week of pregnancy, or normal expected date for the birth. After the twentieth week of pregnancy the fetus is said to be viable. This means it is capable of independent life. However in some cases the fetus may be expelled from the uterus before the thirty-sixth week. These circumstances will bring a patient into accident and emergency. The nurse must remember that obstetric conditions in the accident and emergency department are due to abnormalities generally, although some patients present within the thirty-sixth week of pregnancy with abdominal pain denying that they are pregnant and deliver normally.

Patient Care

For the accident and emergency nurse the care of the pregnant patient means:
1. Position the patient on a trolley.
2. Immediately recognize the condition from:
   The patient's history.
   Spasmodic abdominal pains causing the patient to push down.
   Watery vaginal discharge.
   Appearance of part of the fetus such as the head, feet or the umbilical cord.
3. Immediate notification of the appropriate staff, the midwife and the obstetrician. There should be a midwife available to each accident and emergency department. Ensure that you know the number to ring in your hospital.
4. Reassure the patient.
5. Prepare the equipment that will be required:
   Delivery pack
   Umbilical clamps
   Suction apparatus

REVISION OBJECTIVES

1. List the characteristic signs and symptoms of an acute abdominal condition and the possible causes.
2. Describe the patient care and importance of observations for an acute abdominal condition.
3. Explain the care of a patient in the X-ray department.
4. Define the term ectopic pregnancy and describe the care in order of priority.
5. Outline and annotate common obstetric conditions and their related care.

11
Violence and Major Disasters

VIOLENT INJURIES

Violence can be defined as a vehement or destructive exertion of physical force. Unfortunately, violent behaviour in patients is becoming an increasing problem in the accident and emergency department. Also the results of violent, unlawful behaviour in the community are presenting more patients to the accident and emergency department who have been victims of:
    Traumatic injuries (see Chapter 8)
    Rape
    Child abuse
    Wife battering
    Granny battering

Violence Within the Department

Violence within the department may come from the patient or the person or people accompanying the patient. It more commonly occurs on Friday and Saturday nights in Britain and is largely due to the influence of alcohol. Another cause of violence can be frustration at long waiting periods for treatment. Unfortunately, the attitude of the accident and emergency staff, often quite innocent but due to extreme pressure of work, may provoke violent behaviour.
Note. It is important that
    The violent person is protected from self-injury.
    Staff and people within the department are protected from the violent person.

Prevention

The first priority — to try to prevent any or further violent behaviour — is sometimes extremely difficult. A person may appear to be calm and normal at one minute and at the next violence occurs without warning. For example, two incidents encountered in an accident and emergency department were:

A man walked into the department at about 7 a.m. one morning with a nose bleed. He was left with a thermometer while the nurse recorded her observations on his condition and history. Before the nurse had time to make notes, however, the patient threw the thermometer into the air and started 'wrestling' with his chair which would, no doubt, have followed the thermometer had it not been bolted to the floor. He stormed out of the department without further treatment, screaming abuse at all around.

A doctor, engrossed in taking the blood pressure of a patient who was unconscious when admitted and unaware that the patient regained consciousness, did not see the fist which gave him a smashing right hook. The doctor was knocked to the ground and was extremely shaken by the incident.

These incidents briefly illustrate that violence is difficult to prevent on account of its unpredictability. However, there are precautions which should be taken:
1   Give careful explanations, especially if there are long waiting periods involved.
2   Give repeated explanations. Patients' or relatives' attention and understanding may be altered due to their anxiety meaning that they require more explanations.
3   Allow patients to have one relative or friend waiting with them in the department when convenient.
4   Answer questions in a calm, confident manner.
5   Explain rules and regulations when necessary.

Uncontrolled violent situations may be prevented by
1   Alertness to impending problems, e.g., seeking help for arguments between several people in the waiting room which cannot be resolved by staff intervention.
2   Alerting sufficient help to control the situation. Some hospitals are fortunate enough to have security personnel in the accident and emergency department who are able to control a violent outburst. Ambulance personnel, if within the department, are very willing and capable of controlling violence.

Police may have to be called to control the situation. Ensure that you have the telephone number of your local police station.

Conclusions:
1 When possible be aware of impending violence.
2 Call for sufficient assistance to control the situation.
3 Protect the patient and yourself.

Patient Protection

Unfortunately, many patients are unintentionally violent. The disturbed behaviour of the patient may be due to:
   Excess alcohol
   Hypoglycaemia
   Epilepsy
   Mental subnormality
   Psychiatric disturbance

Protecting the patient means ensuring that he or she is in safe surroundings and will not inflict self-injury. It may be necessary to nurse the patient on the floor in an empty cubicle, using pillows for protection. Alternatively, several people may be required to restrain the patient, that is, to hold the patient as still as possible without causing injury. The best way requires 4 people working together to place the patient on a trolley with 2 people to hold the shoulders and wrists down and 2 to hold the knees and ankles.

If the cause of the violent behaviour is hypoglycaemia the patient will require treatment to correct the condition. In other cases the doctor may order tranquillizers or sedatives to control the patient's behaviour.

Staff Protection

For protection always ensure that there are enough members of staff on hand to control the situation. If a patient has to undergo a gastric lavage for the treatment of poisoning, arrange for at least three members of staff to assist in the procedure. The gastric lavage is an unpleasant procedure and many patients object violently during the procedure.

Be aware of the potentially violent patient. Always:
1 Face the patient.
2 Be able to step away from the patient at any time.

3   Always stand between the door and the patient.
4   Ensure that there is help available.
5   Talk in a calm voice and explain all procedures.

The Unco-operative Patient

Even patients who have brought themselves into the accident and emergency department may be unco-operative and refuse the treatment prescribed by the doctor. To obtain a patient's co-operation can often become a time-consuming task. The nurse calmly explains the treatment and asks for the patient's co-operation; if this is not forthcoming, do not continue to persuade, ask for the help of the nurse in charge or a doctor. A patient will sometimes heed the advice of the senior nurse or a doctor. If the patient remains adamant and will still not agree to treatment, then he or she must be asked to sign a form stating that medical treatment has been refused and that the patient is responsible for his or her own medical condition. A patient, cannot be forced to sign the form and may leave the department without further treatment and without signing the form.

Consent for Treatment

Consent is not needed from:
  Children under 16 years of age, **but** parental or a guardian's consent is needed for care to be given.
  Patients who may be a danger to themselves or others. These patients may be retained in hospital under the Mental Health Act (England and Wales).

Violence within the Community

When violence occurs within the community causing injury, observations and the taking of the history of these patients are extremely important as they may be used in a court of law.

Rape

Rape is a sexual assault on a male or female. Victims of rape may go directly to a police station where the police surgeon will be responsible for the examination. Some rape victims, however, come directly to the accident and emergency department of a hospital.

In the accident and emergency department the important initial care is to observe the patient and to leave the patient's clothing in place. There may be other injuries which require immediate treatment, if so treatment must be commenced immediately.

The police surgeon should be contacted. Generally in the United Kingdom, the police surgeon accompanied by a police woman, in the case of a female victim, will come and examine the patient. It is important that accurate information is taken in case it is necessary for treatment to remove the patient's clothing. If the clothing must be removed it must be observed for signs of violence and semen stains.

It may be necessary for a gynaecologist to examine the female patient.

Special considerations must be given to a rape victim:

Privacy. A closed room is essential for privacy. A curtained cubicle does not allow the patient to give a confidential history.

Emotional support. The patient is generally extremely distressed and will need emotional support. Be ready to listen to and to answer any questions.

Examination. The female patients will have a vaginal examination so the equipment must be prepared. For some patients this examination is extremely distressing as the experience of the rape assault is still fresh in their minds so careful explanations of the procedure and its importance are essential. If the police woman is not present a female nurse **must stay** with the patient.

For some patients the procedure is painful due to the trauma inflicted during the rape. The doctor must decide whether the patient requires analgesia or sedatives. The taking of the history and the subsequent examination can be very time-consuming so check with the doctor whether the patient can have anything by mouth and, if it is allowed, offer the patient a cup of tea.

Do not leave the patient alone in the department. Ask the patient if the next of kin is to be informed and do so only if the patient wishes.

Child Abuse

Children can enter the accident and emergency department with a variety of traumatic injuries. The nurse be alert to:
1   Those children who seem to have repeated injuries.
2   Those children whose injuries do not seem to coincide with the history of the incident, e.g., it is unusual for a child to sustain a fractured femur after tripping over the carpet.
3   The parent who is hostile and aggressive.
4   The account of the incident which varies from one parent to another.
5   The child who is extremely withdrawn and possibly showing signs of neglect in clothing, diet and hygiene.

There should be a list kept in each department of children who have repeated injuries and who could be victims of child abuse.

If you suspect child abuse:
1   Undress the child completely as the doctor will need to make a thorough examination. Observe the child.
2   Talk normally to the child and parents or guardian and obtain a history of the incident. Do not in any way indicate that you suspect child abuse.
3   Report your findings to the doctor (paediatrician) before the child is seen. Some cases of child abuse may require immediate resuscitation. Ensure that you have summoned help. The case may be discussed as soon as the child's condition is stable.
4   The child may be admitted to hospital for a 24 – 28 hour period of observation.
5   Social services and health visitors must be notified as the child will require a careful follow-up after discharge.

As child abuse is unlawful all written records concerning the child must be completed accurately as they may be used in a court of law.

Battering

Battering is physical abuse which can result in serious injury. Whatever the injury the patient must be first treated for that injury (see Chapter 4).

The Battered Husband or Wife. The battered husband or wife often comes to the department alone. Usually, the patient does not know whether to return home and does not know where else to go. The patient will only be admitted to hospital if the physical condition warrants admission, so it may be necessary to contact the social services department in order to ensure that the patient has somewhere to go when leaving the hospital.

The injuries should be carefully documented as the patient may wish to take legal action against the other partner. Whether legal action is taken is the decision of the patient and the nurse must not attempt to make these decisions for the patient.

Treat the injuries, listen to the problems and give assistance when requested, even if the patient insists on returning home where he or she may be further ill-treated.

Legal advice may be arranged through the social services department.

The Battered Granny or Elderly Person. The battered granny or elderly person is the victim of physical abuse often from a robbery attempt, but also may have received the injury from a relative. Apart from physical injuries, he or she may be shocked and frightened due to the degree of violence of the attack. If 'parent battering' is suspected, follow with appropriate modifications the steps recommended for suspected child abuse. Whenever possible stay with the patient in the department, reassure the patient and explain the care and treatment which will be given.

Unfortunately many of these injuries require the patient to be admitted to hospital for treatment so ensure that the next of kin is informed. The police may be asked to inform the next of kin, who may also be elderly.

The police will need information concerning the robbery or the abuse or both but this is not the responsibility of the nurse to impart this information (see Chapter 2). The doctor must be consulted. The doctor will speak to the police or let the police talk with the patient if the patient's condition is satisfactory.

If the police see the patient in the department allow them privacy in which to take the statement but do not allow the patient to become tired or distressed. Return to check on the patient's condition within 5 minutes.

General Advice. In all of these incidents of violence in the community it is the nurse's role to inform the doctor of any relevant information and to document carefully any important observations and treatment.

All patients are entitled to confidentiality so do not discuss their condition or care with anyone except the nursing staff and the doctor on duty at the time.

The police must be allowed access to the patient when the condition of the patient is stable as the police have a report to compile.

Newspaper reporters should be referred to the hospital administration for an official report on the patient (see Chapter 2). The nurse must never give out any information to reporters.

MAJOR DISASTERS

A major disaster is an incident from any cause that involves several people and necessitates the activity of several emergency services. It results in an emergency call, e.g., involving police, ambulance, fire and other services.

A disaster will affect each accident and emergency department differently because of the size and staffing level of each department. Each department should have a hospital policy to deal with major disasters. Make yourself familiar with the policy and with the location of emergency equipment for a disaster.

Disaster policies aim to give a high standard of care to all casualties, treating those in most urgent need first. Priorities must be set.

Priorities

The setting of priorities can begin at the scene of the disaster. Some hospitals may dispatch doctors and nurses to the scene of the disaster. Their function is to assess each casualty and decide which patients require urgent treatment. This is either commenced at the site or on immediate transfer to hospital.

If medical staff are not present at the scene then assessment and the setting of priorities will be commenced immediately as the casualties arrive at the department.

Your hospital policy will state which medical or nursing staff are involved in the initial assessment. The sudden arrival of several casualties in an accident and emergency department should not lead to confusion if staff are aware of the hospital policy and abide by its divisions of work.

The hospital will have received a phone call concerning the disaster, usually before the first casualties arrive. This enables various facilities to be prepared.

Preparation

Preparation for receiving the injured:
1 Telephone communication is important as extra staff may be required.
2 Various areas within the hospital will have to be prepared. Areas will be prepared to receive:
> The acutely ill — usually in the accident and emergency department, so that treatment may be commenced immediately.
> Those who will require treatment as soon as possible. In some hospitals a ward area may be cleared for these patients. In this case the ward must be notified to allow time to move existing patients to another area.
> The walking wounded — this may be an out patients' waiting area.

3 The operating theatres must be prepared and necessary staff members available.
4 Radiography staff must be alerted and necessary staff available.

Other Services

The hospital administrator will be responsible to ensure that other services are available. This will include:

Clerical staff. With the sudden arrival of many casualties it may be impossible for the clerical staff to obtain all necessary clerical information immediately (see Chapter 2). However, patients must be identified. This may be carried out by numbering the patients as they arrive, and placing an identification bracelet on the patient with the number. It is also essential to maintain a register of the patients, their condition, their location in the areas of treatment and the eventual outcome of their condition: discharge or admission. This list must be available to enable the hospital administrator to answer the many phone calls from concerned relatives and friends.

Hospital porters.

Pharmacist. There will be a pharmacist on call who will be able to dispense drugs for patients to take home and to provide extra supplies for the casualties being treated in the hospital.

Laboratory technicians, who must be prepared to receive emergency blood specimens and to cross-match blood. The blood bank technicians must make available units of blood ready for use.

REVISION OBJECTIVES

1 Describe a possible violent situation and ways to prevent or deal with the situation.
2 Outline the ways to recognize cases of abuse and battery.
3 Detail patient care for conditions which result from violence in the community.
4 List the services which are available to respond to a major disaster.
5 Describe hospital policy to deal with major disasters.

Bibliography

Bradley D. (1980) *Accident and Emergency Nursing*. London, Baillière Tindall.
Caroline N.L. (1982) *Emergency Care in the Streets*, 2nd ed. Boston, Little, Brown.
Goulding R. & Vale A. (1979) *A Concise Guide to the Management of Poisoning*. Basingstoke, Dista Products.
Matthew H. & Lawson A.A.H. (1975) *Treatment of Common Acute Poisoning*. Edinburgh, Churchill Livingstone.
Ross J.S. & Wilson K.J.W. (1981) *Foundations of Anatomy and Physiology*, 5th ed. Edinburgh, Churchill Livingstone.
Rutherford W.H., Nelson P.G., Weston P.A.M. & Wilson D.H. (1980) *Accident and Emergency Medicine*. Tunbridge Wells, Pitman Medical.
Skeet M. (1981) *Emergency Procedures and First Aid for Nurses*. Oxford, Blackwell Scientific Publications.

Index

Abdomen
  acute conditions 261-8
    causes 261-2
    diagnostic tests 264-6
    patient care and
      assessment 262-4
    signs and symptoms 261
  inflammation 266, 267
  injuries 203-11
    causes 204
    patient assessment 205-6
    patient care 206-7
  lower, injuries 208-11
Abduction, leg fractures 212
Abortion 270-3
  classification 270
  criminal 271, 272
  incomplete 270, 272
  induced 271-3
  inevitable 270, 272
  spontaneous 270, 272
  therapeutic 271
  treatment 272-3
Abrasions 69-70, 143-4
  corneal 102
Abscesses 72-3
  dressing and patient care 76-7
  incision and drainage
    equipment 73
Accident and emergency
  department
  attendance profile 2
  equipment 3-5
  functions 1
  general advice 9
  health and safety 11-14
  layout 3
  treatment procedures 6
Acetabulum 233
Acidosis, metabolic 47, 173
Adrenaline
  in asthma 138
  in cardiac asystole 48
  in vasoconstriction 55
Agranulocytes 68

Airway
  assessment 22
  clearance 38-40
  intubation 40
  obstruction by the tongue 38-9
  see also Breathing
Alcohol
  and violence 275, 277
  poisoning 189
Ambu bag 4, 42
Ambulance personnel
  communication 7
  controlling violence 276
  history of patient's
    condition 181
  lifting patients 10
Aminophylline
  in asthma 138
  respiratory effects 49, 114, 138
Amylase, serum, pancreatic disease
  265
Anaemia, hypochromic, burns 151
Anaesthesia
  general 73-7
    administration 74-5
    fracture reduction 219-20
    postoperative care 75-7
    preoperative care 73-4
    stages 74-5
  local, fracture care 217-18
Analgesia
  for abscesses 73
  for shock 55
Aneurysm, abdominal 267
Angina 108
  glyceryl trinitrate 113
Ankle, fractures 240-1
  immobilization 215-16
Antibiotics, minor injuries 80
Antigens, blood group 53
Appendicitis 264
Appendix, pain radiation 29
Arachnoid 162
Arm, fractures 230-1
Arrhythmias, cardiac 117-23

Artery, structure and
 disorders 107-8
Aseptic technique 71
Aspartate transaminase
 (ASPT) 112
Asthma 136-9
 intravenous therapy 139
 treatment 137-9
Asystole, cardiac 48, 119, 123
Atheroma, coronary 107
Atrial fibrillation 119-20
Atrio-ventricular node 114-15
Atropine, heart rate effects 48
Autonomic nervous system 155-6

Babinski's sign 179
Bandages
 collar and cuff 90
 figure of eight 220-2
 finger splint 86
 gypsona, preparation 241-2
 ring strapping 87
 Robert Jones 91
 sling 91
 strapping 91
 supportive 85-94
 thumb spica 85
Barbiturates, poisoning 190
Basal ganglia, functions 158
Battering 280-2
 nurse's care role 282
Bleach, poisoning 187-90
Blood clotting 66-7
Blood gases, estimation 43
Blood groups 52-4
 cross-matching 53
Blood pressure 50
Blood tests
 abdominal conditions 265
 myocardial infarction 112
Blood transfusion 52
Blood see also Circulation;
 Haemorrhage
Body temperature see
 Temperature
Bradycardia 51, 113, 120, 164
Brain stem 157, 159-60
 reticular formation 155
Breathing
 air composition 42, 135
 air movement 41
 assessment 22, 41-5
 chest movement 41
 Cheyne-Stokes 132
 difficulties 45

 drugs 49
 intermittent positive
  pressure 138
 mechanism 133-6
 observations 43-5
 rate 44
 voluntary control 134-5
 see also under Respiratory
Bronchitis 139-41
Brook's airway 41
Buer block 217
Bullet wounds 198, 204-5
Bundle of His 115
Burns 143-4, 148-54
 and anaemia 151
 area and depth 149-50
 aseptic technique 71-2
 chemical 152
 eyes 99-101
 electrical 152
 infection and deformity
  prevention 151-2
 minor 70-2
  first aid 70
 psychological care 153-4
Butterfly suture 63

Calcium chloride 48, 49
Calculi, renal 263
Carbon monoxide,
 poisoning 190-1
Cardiac arrest 45-51
 asystole 119, 123
 drugs 48-9
 heart action 48
Cardiac tamponade 199
Cardiac see also under Heart
Carotid pulse 45
Catheterization, in burns 152
Central nervous system 156-60
Cerebellum 157, 159
Cerebral vascular accident 178-81
 signs and symptoms 178-80
 treatment 180-1
Cerebral vascular disorder 177-81
Cerebrospinal fluid,
 rhinorrhoea 99, 165
Cerebrum 156-9
 lobes, functions 157-8
Chemical burns 152
Chest
 drainage 203
 flail 223, 225
 injuries 197-203
Cheyne-Stokes respiration 132

287

Children
    consent for treatment   21-2, 278
    febrile convulsions   172
    non-accidental injuries   280
    pain location   28
    toys   33-4
Chloramphenicol, eye drops   102
Cholecystitis   266
Circle of Willis   177
Circulation
    assessment   22-3, 42, 50-1
    disorders   45-55
    impairment, limb injuries   247-8
    patient care   54-5
Clavicle, fracture   220-2
    immobilization   214, 220-2
Clostridium tetani toxoid   81
Collagen, and wound healing   65
Colles's fracture   214, 222-3
    plaster cast   252-4
    slab application   249-52
Coma, diabetic   175
Complaints, by patients   17-19
Confidentiality   15-17
Congestive cardiac failure   127-9
Consciousness
    assessment   23-6
    regaining, patient care   57-8
    see also Unconsciousness
Consent for treatment   21-2, 73, 278
Continence, control   159-60
Convulsions   171-2
    eclampsia and   273
    see also Epilepsy
Cornea, abrasions   102
Coronary arteries   106-14
Coronary thrombosis *see* Myocardial infarction
Crutches
    fitting and instructions on use   95-7
    following application of leg plaster   258
Cyanosis   22

Death
    cardiac arrest   49-50
    and relatives   35, 50
Defibrillation, cardiac   122
Deformities, fractures and   212
Dermis   143-4
Dexamethasone   57
Diabetes mellitus   172-6
Diabetic ketoacidosis   173

Diazepam   49
    intravenous, fracture reduction   218-19
Digoxin
    heart rate effects   49
    myocardial infarction   113
Disasters   282-4
    non-accident staff help   283-4
    preparation for casualties   283
    priorities   282
Discharging of patients
    eye injuries   103-4
    head injuries   165-6
    minor injuries   83-4
Disc lesions   226
Dislocation
    hip   233-4
    patella   235
    shoulder   232-3
Diverticulitis   266, 267
Documentation   19, 20-2
Domette bandage   91
Dopamine hydrochloride, heart rate effects   48
Dressings   77-80
    finger   77-9
    patient instructions   79-80, 82
Drugs
    cardiac arrest   48-9
    mydriatic   104
Dura mater   162
Dyspnoea   22, 45
Dysuria, lower abdominal injuries   210

ECG (electrocardiogram)   111-12, 116-17
Eclampsia   273
Ectopic heart beats   118, 121
Ectopic pregnancy   268-9
EEG (electroencephalogram)   166
Elderly, battering   281-2
Electrical burns   152
Embolism   107, 108
    cerebral   178
Emergencies, assessment and management   38-59
    see also Disasters
Emphysema, subcutaneous   201
Endocardium   106
Endotracheal tube   40
Entonox   73, 219-20
Enzymes, serum, myocardial infarction   112
Epidermis   142-3

Epilepsy 166-71
 and violence 277
 classification 167-71
 phases 169-71
 treatment 171
 see also Convulsions
Epistaxis (nose bleed) 97-9
 treatment 98-9
Epithelium, squamous 142-3
Equipment 3-5
 emergency 4-5, 40, 45-6
 investigation 5
 patient assessment 5
 safety 12
Erythrocytes
 agglutination 52-3
 sedimentation rate (ESR) 112
Ethical factors 14-15
 confidentiality 15-17
Ethyl alcohol
 and violence 275, 277
 poisoning 187
Examination, patient
 preparation 32
Exercise, after injury 82
Expiration 134
Eyes
 application of drops 102-3
 chemical burns 99-101
 foreign bodies 101-4
 injuries 99-104, 197
  patient instructions on
   discharge 102-4
 irrigation 102
 pads, visual effects 103-4

Face, injuries 196-7
Febrile convulsions 172
Femur
 fracture, immobilization 214-15
 neck fracture 235-7
 shaft fracture 237-9
  fixed traction 237-8
Fibrin, blood clotting 66
Fibrinogen 66
Fibula, fracture 239-40
 immobilization 215
Figure of eight bandage 220-2
Flail chest 223, 225
Floating ribs 223
Foramen magnum 160
Foreign bodies
 eyes 101-4
 under casts 246
Fractures 211

 definition 84
 healing 216
 immobilization 214-16
 lower limbs 233-41
 minor, care of
  collar and cuff 90
  figure of eight 221-2
  finger splint 86
  ring strapping 87-8
 recognition 211-3
 reduction 216-20
 skull 163
 supracondylar 231
 treatment 213-20
 types 211, 212
 upper limbs 230-3
 see also individual regions
Frontal lobe, functions 158
Frusemide 49, 57

Gall-bladder, pain radiation 28
Gastric lavage
 in poisoning 184-6
 preparation and
  procedure 185-6
General anaesthetic 73-5, 219
Glucosuria 174
Glutamic oxaloacetic transaminase
  (SGOT) 112
Glyceryl trinitrate, angina 113
Grand mal 168-71
 phases 168-71
Granulocytes 68-9
Gynaecological disorders 268-74
Gypsona bandage,
  preparation 241-2

Haematemesis 51, 52, 210, 263
Haematuria 51
 lower abdominal injuries 210
Haemolysis 53
Haemoptysis 51-2
Haemorrhage
 abdominal 267
 cerebral 177-8
 control 52
 external 67
  pressure control 63-4
  principles of care 54
  signs 22-3, 51
 internal, signs 22-3, 51
Haemothorax 201-3, 224
Hair follicles 143
Head
 injuries 162-6, 196-7

effects 164
 treatment 164-6
 structural layers 162
Healing
 first intention 65
 second intention 65
Health and safety,
 departmental 11-14
Heart
 arterial disorders 108-13
 block 120-1
 conduction mechanism 114
 injuries 197-9
 layers 106
 muscle 114-17
  see also Myocardium
 pain radiation 28
 rhythm alterations 117-23
 structure 106, 123
 see also under Cardiac
Heat exhaustion 144-5
Heat stroke 146
Heimlich procedure, airway
 clearance 38-39
Hernia 267
 strangulated 264
Hip
 dislocation 233-4
 fractures 209-10
House fire 153
Humerus, fracture 231
Husband battering 280-1
Hydrocortisone 49, 139
Hydroxybutyrate dehydrogenase
 (HBD) 112
Hyperglycaemia 173-6
Hyperkalaemia 175
Hypertension 50
 effects on ventricles 124
Hyperventilation 133, 135
Hypocalcaemia, burns 151
Hypoglycaemia 176-7
 and violence 277
Hypokalaemia 175
 burns 151
Hypotension 50
 left ventricular failure 124
 myocardial infarction 109
Hypothalamus, and
 temperature 27, 28, 145, 159
Hypothermia 27, 146-8
 femoral neck fracture and 235
Hypoventilation 132
Hypoxia 44

Incisions 61-5
 suturing 62-3
Infection, prevention 80-3
Inflammation, abdominal 266, 267
Inflammatory reaction 68-9
Injuries
 minor 61-105
  infection prevention 80-2
  patient instructions 82
 violent 275-82
 see also Trauma; Wounds and
  various organs and regions
Inspiration
 changes after injury 200-2
 normal 133-4
Intervertebral discs 226
 prolapse 226
Intestine
 nerve damage 267-8
 obstruction 267-8
Intracranial pressure, raised 50, 57
Intubation 40
Intussusception 267
Investigations, nurses' role 5-6
IPPB (intermittent positive
 pressure breathing) 138
Iron, poisoning 191-2
Ischaemia, abdominal 264
Isoprenaline, heart rate effects 48

Jacksonian epilepsy 168
Jaw, fractures 197
Jugular vein 128

Keratin 143
Ketoacidosis, diabetic 173, 175
Ketonuria 173
Kidneys, calculi 263

Laburnum seeds, poisoning 192
Lacerations 61-5
Lactic dehydrogenase (LDH) 112
Laparotomy, abdominal
 injuries 207
Left ventricular failure 123-7
Leg, abduction 212
Leucocytes
 bacterial reaction 68-9
 count, myocardial infarction 112
Lifting and moving,
 patients 9-11, 13, 14
Lignocaine hydrochloride, heart
 rate effects 48, 113

Limbs
  injuries 230-41
    power loss after 247
  lower, injuries 233-40
  upper, fractures 230-1
Local anaesthetic 217-8
Lost property, procedures 18
Lower limb injuries 233-41
Lund and Browder burn
  charts 149
Lungs
  congestion, left ventricular
    failure 125, 126
  injuries 199-203

Major disasters 282-4
McBurney's point 28
Medicolegal factors 14-15, 16-17, 19
  see also Complaints; Police
Medulla oblongata
  functions 160
  respiratory centre 131
Melaena 51, 210, 263
Melanin 143
Meninges, injuries 163
Mental subnormality, and
  violence 277
Metabolic acidosis
  cardiac arrest 47
  diabetes 173
Monocytes, and bacteria 69
Morphine
  in myocardial infarction 114
  poisoning 192
Myocardial infarction 108-13
  diagnostic tests 111-12, 116-17
  drugs 112-14
  patient history 111
  signs and symptoms 109
  treatment, immediate 110-11
Myocardium 106
  conduction mechanism 106, 114-5
Myxoedema, hypothermia 146

Nerve blocks 59
Nerves, spinal 226-7
Nervous system 155-60
Netalast dressings 77-8
Neutrophils, and bacteria 68-9
Newspaper reporters, and
  nurse 17, 282
Nose bleeds 97-9
Nurse
  communication 6-8

confidentiality 15-6
correct treatment 15, 18
liaison role 6-8, 34-6, 282
psychological role 153-4
role in accident and emergency
  1, 2-10
role in investigations 5
role when patient admitted 6
tact 15
treatment procedures 6

Observations, nurses' role 30-1
Obstetric emergencies 273-4
Obstruction, abdominal 267-8
Occipital lobe, sight and 158
Oculomotor nerves 25, 26
Odour detection 31
Oedema
  cerebral 57
  pulmonary, left ventricular
    failure 125, 126
Oxygen
  Ambu bag 42
  in asthma 138
  inadequate exchange signs 44-5
  masks 44
  precautions 45

P wave, ECG 116
Padding, plaster casts 241
Pain 58-9
  abdominal 206, 263-4
  assessment 27-30
  associated problems 59
  causes 28
    removal 59
  intermittent 29
  radiation 28-9
  relief 58-9
    drugs 59
  severe intractable 29
  sites 28
  thalamus role 157, 158
  types 29
  see also individual organs
Pancreas, disease, serum
  amylase 265
Pancreatitis 266
Paracetamol, poisoning 192-3
Paralytic ileus 267
Parasympathetic nervous
  system 25, 106, 156
Parent battering 281
Parietal lobe, sensations and 157
Patella, dislocation 235

291

Patients
  admission to hospital 6
  assessment 20-1
  belongings 32
  care 31-2
  complaints by 17-19
  discharge 83-4
  general observations 30-1
  lifting and moving 9-11
  protection 277
  reception 20-2
  unco-operative 278
Pelvis
  contents 208
  fractures 208, 209-10
    immobilization 214
  injuries, 208, 229-30
Pericardium 106
Peripheral nervous system 156
Peritonitis 210, 264
Petit mal 168
Pia mater 162
Plaster casts 241-60
  below-knee 256-60
  circulation impairment 247-8
  complications 245-7
  patient instructions 244-5, 248-9, 259-60
  preparation 242-3
  wet, care 244
Platelets 66
Pneumothorax 200, 201-3, 224
  spontaneous 201, 202
  tension 202
Poisoning 181-94
  corrosives 183
  determinants and history 181-2
  noncorrosives 183, 184
  systemic effects 188-9
Police, nurse cooperation 16-17, 282
Polyurea 173
Positioning 11
  in various conditions 31-2
Potassium, muscle activity and 175
Pott's fracture 215-16, 240-1
Practolol, heart rate effects 49
Pregnancy
  complications 270-2
  eclampsia 273
  ectopic 268-9
    psychological aspects 269
  emergencies 273-4

patient care 274
Preoperative care 73-5
Procainamide, heart rate effects 49
Property, patient, care 32-4
  see also Lost property
Prothrombin 66
Psychiatric disorders, and violence 277
Pulse
  in myocardial infarction 109
  rate 50-1
  see also Carotid pulse
Pulmonary oedema 126
Puncture wounds 68-9
Pupil reactions 24-6
Purkinje fibres, ventricular 115
Pyrexia 27

QRS complex, ECG 117

Rape 278-9
Reception, patients 20-2
Reflex actions 155
Relatives
  bereaved 35, 50
  liaison 8, 16, 34-5
  management 16, 35-6
Religion, and death 35
Respiration see Breathing
Respiratory centre 131-6
Respiratory function, changes 131-3
Resuscitation 41-2, 46-7
  fractures and 213
  outcome 49-50
Rhesus factor 53-4
Rhinorrhoea 99
Ribs
  floating 223
  fracture 223-5
    immobilization 214
Ring strapping 87-8
Robert Jones bandage 91-2

Safety
  departmental 11-14
  equipment 12
  patients 12-13
Salbutamol, respiratory effects 49
Salicylates, poisoning 193-4
Salpingectomy, ectopic pregnancy 269
Salpingitis 266, 270
Scalp, injuries 163

Scaphoid fracture 223
Sebaceous glands 143
Sedation, in fracture care 217
Seizures *see* Convulsions; Epilepsy
Sensation, cerebral lobes and 157-9
Serum enzymes 112
Shock
  abortion and 271
  analgesia 55
  anaphylactic (vasodilative) 23, 55
  burns and 150-1
  cardiogenic 23, 54-5
  effects 55
  hypovolaemic 55
  types of 23
Shoulder, dislocation 232-3
Sight, occipital lobe and 158
Sinoatrial node 114-15
Skin, functions 144-8
    see also Abrasions; Burns; Lacerations
  structure 142-4
Skull, fractures 163
Slabs, plaster cast
  Colles's fracture 249-52
  preparation 243-4
Slings 90-4
  collar and cuff 90-1
Spinal cord, injuries 226-7
Spine
  fracture, immobilization 214
  injuries 225-9
    patient care 228-9
    types 226
    vertebrae 225-6
Splints, finger 86-7
Sprains
  definition 84
  treatment 85-97
Staff
  health and safety 14
  protection 277-8
Status asthmaticus 139
Status epilepticus 169
Steristrip dressings 63
Steroids
  asthma 138-9
  cerebral vascular accident 181
Stokes-Adams syndrome 121
Strains
  definition 84
  treatment 85-97
Strapping 88-90

ring 87-8
Stress, and burns 152
Stroke *see* Cerebral vascular accident
Suicide, attempted, by fire 154
Support aids
  crutches 95-7
  walking sticks 94-5
Supracondylar fractures 231
Surgery
  consent 21-2
  positions 10-11
Suturing 62-3
Sweat glands 143
Sympathetic nervous system 25, 106, 156
Synovial joint 233

T wave, ECG 117
Tachycardia 51
  left ventricular failure 124
Temperature 145-8
  normal mechanisms 26-7
  routes of recording 27
Temporal lobe, functions 158
Tetanus, immunization 81-2
Thalamus, functions 157, 158-9
Thomas' splint 238
Thoracotomy, chest injuries 203
Thromboplastin 66
Thrombosis 107, 108
  cerebral 178
  see also Myocardial infarction
Thumb spica 80-1
Thyrotoxicosis 127
Tibia, fracture 239-40
  immobilization 215
Torticollis 226
Tracheostomy, tube 40
Trauma 195-260
Treatment, ethics 15
Tubinette dressings 77-9

Unconsciousness 56-8, 155-61
  advice on discharge 165
  causes 161-2
  effects on reflex actions 155
  observations 24, 56
  see also Coma
Unco-operative patients 278
Upper limb injuries 230-3

Vagus nerve 114
Valium *see* Diazepam
Valuables, care of 33-4

Ventilation, mechanical 42–3
Ventimask 44
Ventricular failure, left,
   acute 123–7
   drugs 127
Ventricular fibrillation 48, 119, 121–2
Vertebrae 225–6
Violence 275–82
   in accident department 275–7
   patient protection 277
   staff protection 277–8
Vitamin D 144
Vitamin K, blood clotting 66
Vitamins A and C 65
Volvulus, intestinal 267
Vomiting, abdominal injuries 210

Waiting, complaints 17–18
Walking aids 94–7
Walking sticks, instructions for
   patient 94–5
Wallace's rule of nine, burn
   area 149
Wife battering 280–1
Wounds
   cleansing 67
   healing 63–4
   inflammatory reactions 65, 68–9
Wrist
   'dinner fork deformity' 222
   fracture 222–4
     immobilization 214
   see also Colles's fracture

X-rays
   abdominal 264–5
   care of patient 265
   skull 165

Zimmer splint 87
Zygote, in ectopic pregnancy 269